"*Fix Your Mood with Food* takes the mystery out of Traditional Chinese Medicine and makes it understandable and accessible. It shows how many people have used it to recover from serious conditions and how you can, too. In our research at the Physicians Committee, we have seen the power of dietary changes. With this engaging and practical book, you will have the tools you need for the best of health."

—*Neal D. Barnard, MD; president,*
Physicians Committee for Responsible
Medicine

"*Fix Your Mood with Food* is my new go-to guide for help with my depression and anxiety. It is an informative, clinical, yet easy-to-follow book to guide you into natural healing. I will be buying this book by the boatload for my friends, and I recommend you do the same."

—*Kim Barnouin, coauthor of* Skinny Bitch

"This smart, interesting, easy-to-read guide will have you healthier and happier than you've ever been. A great synthesis of East meets West, *Fix Your Mood with Food* covers it all."

—*Rory Freedman, coauthor of* Skinny Bitch

"Healthy eating has been a big part of my life since 1970, and I can promise you, it leads to healthy living. *Fix Your Mood with Food* is a great resource for those who want to enjoy a healthy and happy life."

—*Ed Begley Jr., actor and environmentalist*

"As a health and wellness advocate and a believer that food is thy medicine and medicine is thy food, *Fix Your Mood with Food* is a great start."

—*John Salley, former NBA player and sports*
commentator

"You are what you eat! So take out the unknowns and start feeling great by digesting the awesome information, facts, and stories that Heather has served up."

—*David de Rothschild, environmentalist*

"All of my life I've struggled with my eating habits. Eating was a way of forgetting about problems. I grew up trying all diets available, from Atkins to South Beach. It wasn't until I changed to a plant-based diet and learned about greens and super foods and read *Fix Your Mood with Food* that I was finally able to feel healthy, stronger, and younger than ever. I lost forty pounds within my first year of going vegan, and now I have plenty of energy to practice yoga, train at the gym, and ride more than one hundred miles a week on my bike. A plant-based diet has helped me overcome my food addictions, and I highly recommended to everyone an expert like Heather."

—*Marco A. Regil, Mexico's number-one*
television game host

"With 70 percent or more of Americans sentenced to prescription medications and their side effects, we desperately need resources like *Fix Your Mood with Food,* which offers an approach to heal our ailments, rather than bandage them. This is true health care!"

—*Ruby Roth, author of* That's Why We Don't
Eat Animals *and* Vegan Is Love

"*Fix Your Mood with Food* is an amazing guide to viewing our food choices as the key to better health. Heather Lounsbury is a magician when it comes to healing the body, and her approachable demeanor and vast knowledge come across seamlessly in this incredible book. Everyone should pick up a copy and start eating smarter!"

—*Jenny Engel and Heather Goldberg,*
Spork Foods

"If you only have one book on health on your bookshelf, it should be *Fix Your Mood with Food.* Heather lays out a wealth of valuable information in a way that is not only easy to digest (pun intended!) but simple to put into practice. Heather clearly illustrates that food is our medicine while also showing readers exactly how, why, and what to get on that happy path to wellness."

—*Carolyn Scott-Hamilton, The Healthy*
Voyager

FIX YOUR MOOD WITH FOOD

THE
"LIVE NATURAL, LIVE WELL"
Approach to Whole Body Health

Heather Lounsbury, L.Ac.

Guilford, Connecticut
An imprint of Globe Pequot Press

To buy books in quantity for corporate use
or incentives, call **(800) 962-0973**
or e-mail **premiums@GlobePequot.com**.

 skirt! ® is an attitude . . . spirited, independent, outspoken, serious, playful and irreverent, sometimes controversial, always passionate.

skirt! ® is an imprint of Globe Pequot Press.
skirt! ® is a registered trademark of Morris Publishing Group, LLC, and is used with express permission.

Illustrations on pp. 13, 22, 39, and 41 courtesy of Shutterstock.com.

Project Editor: Lauren Brancato
Layout Artist: Mary Ballachino
Text Design: Sheryl Kober

Library of Congress Cataloging-in-Publication Data is available on file.

ISBN 978-0-7627-9639-7

Printed in the United States of America

10 9 8 7 6 5 4 3 2 1

The health information expressed in this book is based solely on the personal experience of the author and is not intended as a medical manual. The information should not be used for diagnosis or treatment, or as a substitute for professional medical care.

CONTENTS

The greatest mistake in the treatment of diseases is that there are physicians for the body and physicians for the soul, although the two cannot be separated.

—PLATO

INTRODUCTION

When I was in the tenth grade, I began to question whether doctors were really the authority on the human body. Thanks to a severe case of mononucleosis, I had missed months of school and slept up to twenty hours a day, but the only advice my doctor could give me and my family was to "ride it out." No prescription, dietary advice, or supplement to alleviate symptoms or recover faster—I just had to sit and wait to get healthy. My doctor didn't even recommend vitamin C. Even at fifteen, that didn't sound right. I had also recently given up meat, but I had no clue about how to be a vegetarian, and there weren't many resources back then to guide me. Like most teenagers, I was still eating junk food, just without any meat. I had no idea how to do it right. Again, my doctor seemed to be no help. I decided to be proactive and learn about health and wellness on my own, which eventually led me to Traditional Chinese Medicine (TCM).

I've always been open to different cultures and ways of thinking, thanks to learning other languages and the foreign exchange students my family hosted in our home while I was growing up. The world came to us in the form of guests from Germany, France, Belgium, and El Salvador. A girl from Iran stayed with us for an entire year. The student who made the biggest and most lasting impression on me was a graduate student from China named Shen. One day my younger sister had a cut that just wouldn't stop bleeding. Shen went to his room, returned with a mysterious powder in a jar, and applied it. Instantly, the flow of blood stopped without toxic chemicals or even a Band-Aid. That was the first time—but certainly not the last—I saw an herbal mixture heal an injury. The memory of how Shen used a natural cure stayed with me and ultimately led me down the path to my career as an herbalist and practitioner of TCM.

TCM uses a combination of acupuncture, herbs, and nutrition to heal patients both inside and out. I began my TCM journey by learning massage and acupuncture before attending medical school at the Emperor's College of Traditional Oriental Medicine in Santa Monica, California, which teaches a mix of Western and Chinese medicine. Today I have my own private practice as a licensed acupuncturist and herbalist in California. Many of the principles I employ date back thousands of years; others are more recent techniques created by the people who taught me. I've also created a few techniques of my own, which I've developed both by treating patients and by doing my own research.

Since TCM is just beginning to become mainstream, and there are so many myths out there, I'd like to start with some background to lay the foundation for the theories I will be discussing throughout this book. TCM is a diverse, ancient healing art dating back at least five thousand years. In the late 1990s, a five-thousand-year-old mummy was discovered in the Italian Alps with tattoos of acupuncture points on his body. This discovery suggests that TCM was far-reaching and had been in use long before Marco Polo went to Asia in the late thirteenth century.

The first known written text on Chinese medicine is *The Yellow Emperor's Classic of Medicine*, which dates from approximately 2,500 years ago, around 500 BC. Along with explaining herbs and acupuncture points, this book also discusses philosophy, ecology, astronomy, mathematics, anthropology, and meteorology. It's considered the ultimate manual on how to live life. Most of what is taught and practiced in Chinese medicine today comes from this source, and many of TCM's masters have studied it. Of course, there have been countless books written over the centuries from which to study as well.

TCM originally started when people realized there was a direct link between nature's cycles and the human body's rhythms and cycles. Thousands of years ago people used to take the time to just sit, observe what was going on around them, and contemplate life. There were no smartphones, tablets, video games, or other distractions to keep people from fully experiencing their world. This contemplation led to the development of all the healing modalities practitioners of Chinese medicine use to this day.

Unlike Western medicine, Chinese medicine treats not only the symptoms but also the root cause of any illness or discomfort. This is why it is so effective. If you just treat the symptoms and ignore why you're having a problem, the problem will just keep coming back, or it will manifest in other ways. Sleeping pills are a perfect example. They don't fix insomnia; if you take a pill because you have a hard time falling or staying asleep, the cause will still be there the next night. Sleeping pills don't help you get a really good night's sleep; they just knock you out—plus, the next day most people feel in a sort of hangover. Many become so used to having brain fog and drinking caffeine to force themselves awake that they don't even realize the sleeping pills are the cause of their fatigue and fuzzy head every morning. In addition to not providing the desired result of being truly rested, this course of action doesn't necessarily relieve the underlying stress, which may manifest in many other ways, such as heart disease, high blood pressure, headaches, and more.

TCM looks at why a person has insomnia and how to heal that. That's one of the main reasons I chose to study Chinese medicine in the first place. Why not get to the root of the issue and be rid of the illness once and for all? Is it too much caffeine? Side effects from medication? Hormonal imbalances? High stress levels? Food allergies? TCM practitioners treat the cause instead of prescribing pills to mask the symptoms. Ultimately, the goal is to prevent the sleepless nights from coming back, but balancing your hormones or reducing your stress levels will improve your overall health, not just your sleep. Of course, Western medicine has its benefits when it comes to emergencies, surgery, and broken bones, but, unfortunately, there's not much emphasis on prevention or getting to the cause of an illness. As nutrition, holistic medicine, and TCM become more popular, medical schools are getting on board. Half of all medical schools—including

Harvard, Yale, Johns Hopkins, and UCLA—are now teaching classes on alternative medicine, showing that the medical establishment has grown to accept the value of holistic approaches.

TCM also stems from the idea that our emotions and physical body are inextricably linked. According to TCM, there are five emotions (anger, heartache, sadness, fear, and worry) that lead to physical ailments when suppressed. Simply put, when you keep these feelings inside, your body will become sick on the outside. But TCM goes a step further, linking each emotion to an organ of the body and showing how, by eating specific foods (and avoiding others), you can resolve emotional wounds and their physical manifestations.

If you are new to Eastern medicine and/or TCM, this may sound far-fetched. But I've seen, time and time again, that when emotions aren't dealt with in a healthy manner, they can have negative consequences on the physical body. Nearly all the patients who have visited my clinic have been able to trace their physical symptoms to emotional issues and improper eating habits. And regardless of whether they were emotionally ready for change or not, every single one has had results.

Healing can occur through counseling and therapy, meditation and prayer, or acupuncture and herbal supplements, but for all these avenues, the right foods can also help get you on the road to recovery. I've seen it firsthand. I've had patients who were heartbroken, angry, and sick at our first visit become happy, satisfied, and healthy by our last, simply by changing their diet.

HOW YOU HANDLE STRESS

Everyone has some form of stress in their lives; it's part of being human. It's how you handle that stress that is important. TCM can help you manage your stress and become a more carefree, happy-go-lucky person.

Start by thinking about how you feel on a daily basis. Do your moods fluctuate throughout the day? Would you consider yourself a calm, even-keeled person? Or are you more of a worrywart or a rageaholic?

Do any of the following statements sound familiar?

- I'm depressed a lot.

- I haven't dealt with the death of my spouse.

- I experience road rage whenever I get in the car.

- I have panic attacks that seem to come from nowhere.

- I'm afraid of abandonment, failure, heights, being vulnerable.

- I worry all the time.

- I never seem to laugh.

- I can't let go of the past/that person.

- I get angry for no good reason.

- I'm still angry about something that happened twenty years ago.

Does one of these statements hit you at your core? If so, it may be what I call your *emotional theme*. Most people have a theme to their emotional state. Still not sure? Then keep reading. This book should give you some insights as to what your emotional theme is. I've included several anecdotes and detailed stories about some of my patients to help you figure it out. Reading other people's experiences will help you relate your own.

As you go through this book, you'll see why I consider finding your theme essential for a proper Chinese medicine diagnosis, treatment, and dietary suggestions. If a patient doesn't seem open to sharing, I don't press. But nearly everyone gives me at least some hints about their emotions without even realizing it. They'll mention how they handled a stressful situation at work, how mad they are at their spouse, or how they've been sleeping. Even these simple clues give me the answers I'm looking for. If there's a link to their symptoms, I can deduce what their emotional theme is as well.

"Negative" emotions can be an everyday occurrence. (I put the word *negative* in quotes because I encourage people not to view any emotion as negative, wrong, or bad. All of them are OK. Feeling is part of being alive.) Just the experience of driving to work every morning can bring a whole host of feelings. Have you heard the term *road rage* before? Ever experienced it? Well, come to L.A., where I live, and drive on the freeway at 5:30 on a Friday evening. You'll develop a very deep understanding of the concept.

As a society, we're taught not to really feel or express our emotions. *Be tougher. Boys don't cry. Don't be so sensitive. Being angry is bad. You shouldn't be afraid. Take a pill for that. If you're still sad, something's wrong with you.* These are all messages we learned from family or friends, school, or movies and TV.

Of course, sometimes we're in a social or work situation where it would be pretty awkward to cry or yell. Whatever those feelings are, they need to come out at some point. Processing them later on doesn't usually happen. Ever wonder why you have an emotional outburst for seemingly no reason? It may be from all the times you didn't let off steam.

By not expressing ourselves fully or completely ignoring emotional discomfort, we can make ourselves sick. This has become an epidemic in Western culture. Stuffing feelings down with cigarettes, shopping, sugar, liquor, sex, caffeine, drugs (legal or illegal), or food is not the ideal way to cope. But, unfortunately, with the amount of pressure most of us are under, this has become the norm. Stuffing our faces with cake and ice cream, racking up credit card debt on things we don't need, or binging on booze every weekend gives us a quick fix. But none of these takes away the underlying anxiety or pain.

Sometimes suppressing a memory or feeling is the only way a person can handle a situation. For example, abuse victims often do this as a survival tool. The only way many abused children can handle their horrible experiences is to block them out completely. Most abuse survivors forget at least some of their traumatic experiences just to be able to function in everyday life. It's a coping mechanism that may last for their entire lives.

Your emotions may not be as intense as those of survivors of physical, emotional, or sexual abuse, but if you learn to cope by blocking out or suppressing experiences, the damage can last a lifetime. Whether we come from healthy, functional homes or not, we learn how to deal with and express our feelings by watching our parents and siblings. As adults we carry these learned behaviors with us, at least to some extent. When we are uncomfortable or can't handle an experience or emotion, we consciously or subconsciously don't allow ourselves to feel it.

Even Western medicine is catching up: Several studies have shown a link between suppressing emotion and disease, as well as shown how expressing negative emotions and releasing tension can lead to physical healing—basically, what I practice in a nutshell. This book will give you tools to process the old emotional garbage through simply modifying your eating habits.

You might have been given some great nutritional advice in the past. Your cholesterol levels and your weight may have dropped. But maybe some of your health concerns just won't go away. Or that last ten pounds you need to lose refuses to come off. Those sinus headaches keep coming back. Maybe your health issues haven't been alleviated or even diagnosed with Western medicine. The frustration alone can make you sicker. Why? Holding on to anger or fear can contribute to physical issues. I'm not saying you're at fault, but if you haven't dealt with past hurts and let them go, they will eventually make you sick. Choosing the right foods to support your healing process is also key.

My goal with my patients, and this book, is to show you how to use the ancient practice of TCM to heal your body from the inside out. It's very empowering to be in charge of your own healing, to finally understand what's going on with your moods and your body and, most importantly, know how to fix it. I will give you the information you need to have the same healing experience my patients have enjoyed, from the basics of TCM to learning which foods you should incorporate into your diet or avoid.

Fix Your Mood with Food has four sections. Part I expands on the information I've given in this introduction to explain the fundamentals of TCM. Part II addresses each of the five emotions, their related organs, and foods that can improve them. I'll give you the tools you need to work on your unique individual issues, as well as heal occasional imbalances in your emotional and physical well-being. Don't worry; this isn't a diet book. I'm not going to tell you to only eat kale and wheatgrass—though those are wonderfully healthy foods to put on your grocery list. But I *will* show how decadent foods like coconut whipped cream and creamy broccoli soup can be equally as nourishing. After all, healthy doesn't have to be boring or bland; it can be nutritious and delicious.

I'll also share case studies that illuminate the emotional and physical connection. Though the names and a few minor details have been changed, each case study is the profile of a real person who came to me for help. These experiences were life changing for each and every patient I've profiled, and I hope they will inspire you. Part III includes some Western-based nutritional advice that you can use in conjunction with the more holistic Eastern perspective on food given in Part II. This is where I will share some broad ideas about what constitutes a healthy diet and provide specific guidance on what heals and hurts your body. Part IV sums up the information and leads into the Food, Glorious Food section, which lists a wide variety of healthy food choices.

In the end, I hope this book will help you discover, as I have, how Traditional Chinese Medicine—with a little Western medicine thrown in—can empower you to fix a wide variety of emotional and physical ailments simply through the food you eat.

PART I

Ancient Chinese Secrets Revealed

The superior doctor prevents sickness;
The mediocre doctor attends to impending sickness;
The inferior doctor treats actual sickness.

—CHINESE PROVERB

CHAPTER 1

I Second That Emotion

Traditional Chinese Medicine (TCM) emphasizes the importance of emotions and their role in our physical well-being. Each physical ailment may be caused by an emotional issue or event or vice versa. Because I embrace this more holistic view of the body, I consider my patients' emotions as an important part of the larger picture of their physical health.

You probably learned in high school biology about the functions and locations of all the organs. With this book, you want to try to forget what you've learned (if you haven't already). It is important to establish that, as a practitioner of TCM, when I mention a particular organ—such as the spleen—I am referring to a complex system of connected symptoms and emotions, not an actual body part and its typically related functions. TCM views what we Westerners consider organs as having an energetic and esoteric role in their impact on one's health. Their imbalances might manifest in ways that have nothing to do with the physical organ. There is some overlap in the

3

TCM and Western functions of each organ, but sometimes they're worlds apart. Some organs don't play a role at all in TCM. For example, the appendix and thymus gland are not really considered at all in diagnosing or treating a patient. Sometimes two organs are viewed as one: The adrenal glands are considered to be the same organ as the kidneys (which sort of makes sense, since the adrenals sit right on top of the kidneys).

TCM advocates believe that we're born predisposed to certain weaknesses and imbalances in specific organs. How we live our lives determines whether these problems affect us at all and to what extent. Living a balanced life—including following the tenets of Chinese nutrition and eating organic whole foods, getting enough restful sleep and plenty of exercise, avoiding drugs and overmedicating, having ways to cope with and minimize stress—supports your body's ability to function optimally. In Part II, I will go into greater detail about the relationship between our emotions and our physical health.

Let's use the spleen as an example of how Western medicine views the organ as compared to TCM. Western thought sees the spleen's functions as increasing immunity, storing and releasing blood, producing red blood cells in fetuses, and destroying bacteria and worn-out blood cells. A few health issues related to the spleen are some forms of anemia, elevated white blood cell count, and Hodgkin's disease.

In the view of Chinese medicine, however, the spleen gives energy, or qi, to muscles and organs to move and have strength. It aids digestion of food and drink, converting it into qi and blood. In addition, the spleen keeps blood in the blood vessels, governs your thought process, and prevents prolapse (hemorrhoids are an example of this) and sagging. Some related health issues would be varicose veins, obsessive thinking, weak muscles, and slow metabolism.

In TCM each organ has an emotion or emotions connected to it. When a particular organ is weak, a person will have issues with the emotion related to that organ, and if a person doesn't deal with an emotional problem, this will cause a weakness or imbalance in its respective organ, thus leading to more issues around that particular emotion, creating a vicious cycle. For example, in Chinese terms, someone who worries or habitually overthinks things will usually have a weak spleen, which followers of TCM see as a cause of sugar cravings. Eating sugar, especially refined sugar, weakens the spleen. A weak spleen makes you worry even more, thus craving even more sweets. Unless you cut out soda, processed food, and desserts and learn how to cope with what's worrying you, this pattern can continue for years.

TCM also teaches that each organ is connected to other organs or parts of the body in a very different way than you're used to understanding. For example, in TCM the liver is related to anger, frustration, muscle, and connective tissue. What does this mean? When there's an imbalance in the liver, it can manifest in tight muscles or

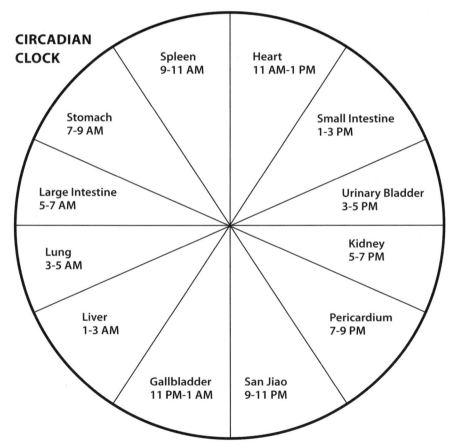

Each organ works its hardest and is most vulnerable during its time slot. Symptoms for a particular organ may be aggravated or only show up during its time frame.

muscle spasms. Another example is the lungs manifest on the skin, so someone with asthma or other breathing issues will most likely have some kind of skin disorder, such as eczema or rashes.

Today in the West, circadian rhythms and the body clock are familiar concepts, often arising in discussions about night-shift workers or cross-country travel. But the Chinese theorized the existence of the circadian clock thousands of years ago: Recorded proof of this theory dates back to Greece during the fourth century BC. It differs from the modern conception of circadian rhythms in that the Chinese had specific two-hour time frames of maximum energy for each organ, whereas the West has come up with physiological functions at their peak without really mentioning specific body parts. Circadian rhythms are relevant to all life, whether animal, plant, or insect. All are influenced by the time of day and amount of light to which they are exposed.

The Chinese circadian clock has many applications in modern life. Here are some examples:

- If you wake up at 4:00 a.m. on a regular basis, you may have some unresolved grief to work out.

- In a given twenty-four-hour period, blood pressure is highest at 6:30 p.m. The kidneys, which are related to the emotions of fear and anxiety, are in charge of that time slot (5:00–7:00 p.m.), and the kidneys regulate blood pressure.

- Your body should have its deepest sleep around 2:00 a.m., but if you have anger issues or problems with your liver, you could be wide awake or having disturbing dreams at that time.

Below are the two-hour increments assigned to each part of the body in TCM.

Lungs 3:00–5:00 a.m.
Large intestine 5:00–7:00 a.m.
Stomach 7:00–9:00 a.m.
Spleen 9:00–11:00 a.m.
Heart 11:00 a.m.–1:00 p.m.

Small intestine 1:00–3:00 p.m.
Bladder 3:00–5:00 p.m.
Kidneys 5:00–7:00 p.m.
*Pericardium 7:00–9:00 p.m.
*San Jiao 9:00–11:00 p.m.
Gallbladder 11:00 p.m.–1:00 a.m.
Liver 1:00–3:00 a.m.

*Note: The two organs identified with asterisks, pericardium and San Jiao, won't be mentioned in future chapters. I've decided to leave them out primarily because they're thought to have the least influence on our physical and mental health, but I will give a brief explanation here. Both are connected to the Fire element. San Jiao, translated as "triple burner," does not exist in Western anatomy and physiology. It is broken up into three levels in the torso. The top includes the chest, lungs, and heart. The middle is below the diaphragm to the belly button. The lowest of the three encompasses the area between your belly button and your bottom. The San Jiao is most responsible for aiding in metabolism of food and fluid and keeping all the organs communicating with each other. The pericardium is the heart protector, in both TCM and Western terms. In TCM it protects the heart physically and emotionally from any harm: Whether defending you from someone yelling or an infection in the blood, a healthy pericardium will make sure the heart can't be injured.

You breathe. You poop. You eat. At least that's how the day should start. If the order gets thrown off balance, you get cranky, tired, or sick. The order of the clock and its influence can be disrupted in many ways. Depression, alcoholism, poor sleep quality and sleeping habits, seasonal affective disorder, bipolar disorder, and jet lag can all throw off your natural body rhythms. Artificial lighting and electricity are both big contributors to compromising this system. (If you can find a way to avoid having electric items in your bedroom and make it as dark as possible while you're sleeping, this will help tremendously.)

You can have a positive impact on your circadian clock. For example, the stomach is most active from 7:00 to 9:00 a.m., so it's the perfect time to get in a nourishing breakfast. You can also use the clock to decide the best times to exercise or get ready for bed. Start paying attention to when you feel your best throughout the day and when you're most tired. This will give you clues as to what organs need some extra TLC.

CHINESE NUTRITION

You might be asking, what is Chinese nutrition? How is it different from Western nutrition? Chinese medicine and nutrition have been around for thousands of years, way before anyone knew what cholesterol, protein, or even vitamin C was. Food wasn't just about survival or taste to the Chinese. Combining the right ingredients to prevent illness and to heal has always been a part of China's culture. The West is only just starting to accept this centuries-old wisdom.

Chinese nutrition is an essential component of TCM, as important as acupuncture or herbal medicine. If you want to use this book to make real changes in your life, you must begin to view food in a completely new way. Each vegetable, grain, fruit, nut, seed, or animal product has an energetic value to it. Everything you eat has an effect on specific organs and yin, yang, qi, and/or blood. Foods can be warming or cooling. They can calm you or get you energized without the sedative quality of booze or the jitteriness of caffeine. In the remaining chapters in Part I, I will explain more about yin and yang, qi, and the other ancient concepts that form the basis for TCM. Later I'll give you lists of delicious, easy-to-find foods to help you cope and heal from any type of emotional distress, whether it's just waking up on the wrong side of the bed or a full-blown panic attack.

Tension is who you think you should be. Relaxation is who you are.

—CHINESE PROVERB

CHAPTER 2

Point Me in the Right Direction

You might be thinking, *Acupuncture? I don't want some old Asian guy sticking five-inch needles all over my body! No thanks.* Yes, there are many misconceptions about acupuncture. Even though more and more people are using it in the West every year, it's still considered pretty weird, and only for Californians like myself. Some consider it New Age or only for hippie types. But that's not the case at all.

Most people assume that acupuncture has to hurt. They typically equate the size of a syringe used for drawing blood to an acupuncture needle. Yet acupuncture needles can be less than one-quarter the width of a syringe. Their thinness has been likened to a strand of hair. Acupuncture needles are so fine that a majority of the time my patients don't feel them going in, and once the needles are inserted, you shouldn't feel them at all. My new patients are always shocked by how easy and painless acupuncture is. In fact, the process of getting acupuncture is so relaxing that virtually all my patients fall asleep for at least a portion of their thirty-minute sessions.

Even if you've had a treatment, you might not know much about it. Many of my patients, who have been coming to me for years and are total believers, don't know about acupuncture's long history or that its effectiveness has been proven through both years of anecdotal evidence and modern scientific studies.

There are several theories on how *acupoints*—the points on the body where needles are inserted—were discovered. The most popular and widely accepted is that their locations and functions were divinely inspired. In China five thousand years ago, it was considered the norm for people to meditate for years, decades, and even entire lifetimes in remote caves and forests. These long periods of meditation were attempts to find the answers to life's questions: how to live life, why we are here, and how to end suffering. The answers were passed on orally from teachers to their students. Some ancient traditions and teachings are still only passed down orally.

Another theory posits that points are based on astronomy, suggesting that there is a direct correlation between the stars and planets and the placement of needles on our bodies. There are acupoints that go along each side of the spine and are located by each of the various vertebrae. These points, discovered thousands of years ago, are used to treat the various internal organs and emotions (depending on location). For example, a point to treat the kidneys and anxiety is level with the lumbar 3 vertebrae and about an inch away from either side of the spine, depending on a person's size. It is now known in Western medicine that there is a nerve at this exact location that stimulates the function of the kidneys. The same can be said for all of the points related to organs along each side of the spine. What's so amazing is that nerve pathways and functions weren't found until centuries after these acupoints were initially used, yet the ancient Greeks, who are known for their medical advances and had only a slight understanding of what nerves were and their role in physiology, somehow knew these precise points were important.

THE POWER OF QI

To understand TCM you must also become acquainted with the concept of qi. *Qi* is a word you might have heard before in a yoga or martial arts class; it's become a part of our vocabulary and is even accepted as a word in Scrabble. But what is it exactly? Qi is the energy or life force of the body. It flows through what are called *energy channels, pathways,* or *meridians,* as explained below.

Even modern science now agrees that qi/energy does exist and flows in particular patterns throughout the body; bioenergetics is an area of biochemistry that studies the flow of energy in living things. All living beings have an electromagnetic energy current. These electrical and magnetic fields are related to lymph and blood flow, nerve conduction, heart and brain function, and many more biological roles.

Without enough qi your organs can't function to their full potential, and your energy levels will be greatly reduced. Qi facilitates moving, protecting, rising, and transforming. When flowing smoothly and unobstructed, qi is in charge of supporting your immune system, keeping organs and body parts operating to their potential, and giving you energy. You can't really have too much qi, but it can become stagnant, perhaps by injury. When qi is stagnant, it can cause a blockage in an organ or area, causing pain, masses, or tumors.

What do I mean by moving, protecting, rising, and transforming? By "moving," I mean literally moving: getting your muscles working, the synapses in your brain connecting, your heart pumping, and blood flowing. Qi gives you energy and the ability to think, jump, run, and even smile.

The qi in your lungs is the main source of support for your immune system. It is in charge of protecting you from illness or pathogens that might enter your body and make you sick. If your lung qi is strong, you'll rarely get sick. When you do get sick, you won't be bedridden and will recover quickly. So qi protects you from harm.

Without enough qi, things begin to sag—sagging being the opposite of rising. Your skin, eyelids, colon (e.g., hemorrhoids), veins (e.g., spider and varicose veins), muscles (e.g., hernias), and uterus can droop or protrude.

The spleen and stomach need adequate amounts of qi from food and drink to transform nutrients into healthy blood and more qi. Someone who doesn't have enough spleen qi may be anemic or experience fatigue. They complain about being exhausted, even if they sat on the couch all day or slept ten hours.

Qi has several origins. An important source of qi is passed from your parents at conception and stored in your kidneys. If your parents have weak qi, they will pass this on to you, making you predisposed to certain illnesses. The quality of their qi can be due to age, lifestyle, eating habits, medications, and the qi passed down by their parents and ancestors. This qi is known as the source qi, or *jing qi* in Chinese. In Western terms, *jing qi* is your genes. Congenital diseases or a predisposition to certain illnesses would be said to come from this qi; for example, if your parents or grandparents had a heart condition or premature gray hair, they might pass that on to you through their *jing qi*.

You can increase your *jing qi* with healthy living. It's definitely not etched in stone that you'll get certain illnesses. All the tips you learn in this book will support and strengthen your source qi.

QI AND DIET

For centuries Chinese medicine has recognized the connection between nutrition and health. Your diet has a large influence on each organ's qi levels, which is one reason why eating the right foods is so important for overall fitness. Some qi comes from food and is created by the spleen. (The Western equivalent would be the idea that vitamins, minerals, and the other nutrients in what you eat become a part of you—"you are what you eat.") Each food has its own function as to which organs it nourishes and how. Oats, dates, kidney beans, apples, cherries, spirulina, and soybeans are all terrific for increasing qi. You will learn more about specific foods and their functions in Chinese terms in Part II. Fast food, processed food, refined sugar, nonorganic food, genetically modified food, extreme diets, soda, alcohol, eating disorders, and binging will all limit and/or deplete the amount of qi you have. Some medications deplete qi by weakening your spleen's ability to make qi as well.

You can also receive qi through certain meditations and exercises. Tai chi, qi gong, and meditation are three traditional ways to gain qi. They help you tap into the abundant qi of the universe. These exercises, common in the East, are becoming increasingly popular in the West as people see the many benefits. Even places like the YMCA offer tai chi classes now.

THE PATHWAYS OF QI

To fully understand the theory behind acupuncture and qi, you must learn about the body's pathways, also known as meridians or channels. The meridians are where the body's energy or qi flows in specific patterns. There are twelve main meridians, ten of which are named after the organs, and two that are related to the yin (Ren or Governing

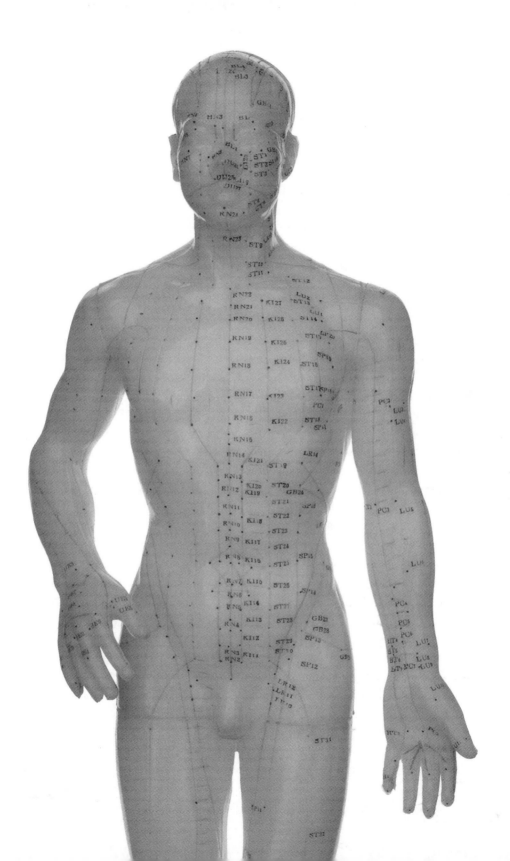

Channel), and yang (Du or Directing Channel) of the body. (You'll learn more about yin and yang in chapter 3.) The ten pathways named after organs are exactly the same on both sides of the body—left and right. There are 362 acupuncture points along these twelve channels. All of them have different functions; some of them have several healing properties. The simplest way to explain this is that acupoints stimulate the flow of qi through the meridians. Don't worry. I won't be quizzing you on this later in the book.

How exactly does qi move through the meridians? Qi flows continually from one meridian to the next in a circuit. This movement initially starts with the first point on the lung channel, then goes to the large intestine channel, and eventually ends up at the liver channel. From there, your qi will then arrive back at the first acupoint along the lung meridian. This is the exact same order shown in the circadian clock mentioned in chapter 1. The process of qi moving through each of the twelve meridians takes twenty-four minutes— two minutes per major channel. Qi flowing through each of the organs takes about twenty-four hours. So receiving acupuncture on the point Large Intestine 4 (LI)—*He Gu* in Chinese, meaning "joining valley"—will stimulate qi from that point until it eventually ends up back at *He Gu* twenty-four minutes later. It is vital that qi constantly flows smoothly for health and well-being. Any obstruction or weakening of the pathways negatively affects your constitution, leading to illness, pain, and/or emotional imbalance.

Those of you who have experienced acupuncture or understand a little bit about it might know about the point Large Intestine 4, located between the thumb and index finger in the meaty part of the hand. This point is tender to the touch on most of my patients due a blockage of qi there.

People often tell me that they've heard pressing this area is helpful to relieve headaches, and it is. But acupuncture to this point also treats anything to do with the face: nasal congestion, skin disorders, toothaches, Bell's palsy, and muscle twitching. It also helps with pain anywhere in the body, and can help relieve a cold, alleviate constipation, and reduce stress. So this point can help pretty much everyone. Because *He Gu* has so many functions, it's probably the most frequently used point. The only time it should not be used is when a woman is pregnant.

Another point that is used quite a lot is called *Yin Tang*. It's located between your eyebrows. Accessing *Yin Tang* is incredibly powerful for calming and reducing anxiety. You can rub it lightly yourself with a fingertip or anoint it with some lavender oil if you're having a tough day or difficulty falling asleep. This point is wonderful for babies who are crying a lot or refusing to go to sleep. They usually respond immediately to the calming effect of *Yin Tang*. Since most of my patients experience high levels of stress, I use *Yin Tang* in a majority of treatments.

Yin Tang is also known as the third eye. This means it helps tap into your intuition. If you've ever taken a yoga or tai chi class, the instructor may have mentioned it as there are a few yoga poses that stimulate this point as well. An example is the child's pose, a resting pose that also encourages circulation in your internal organs.

There's scientific evidence that proves acupoints really do something. It's not just a weird concept thought up by hermits thousands of years ago. Magnetic resonance imaging (MRI) of the brain shows that acupuncture points have an effect on brain function: When a needle is inserted into a specific point, the brain lights up in the exact place where the brain controls that function.

I'll give you a couple of examples. A point on the foot called Liver 3, or *Tai Chong* ("great rushing"), is used to treat eye disorders. When Liver 3 was needled in a study, the middle occipital gyrus, an area related to the visual cortex or your vision and eyes, was activated and lit up in MRIs. So Western medicine agrees that a point on your foot stimulates the part of your brain in charge of vision. Three points used in combination to treat migraines and headaches—Gallbladder 34, or *Yang Ling Quan* ("yang hill spring"), Gallbladder 20, or *Feng Qi* ("wind pool"), and San Jiao 5, or *Wai Guan* ("outer pass")—have likewise been proven to stimulate specific brain regions associated with reducing pain. Pretty amazing, right?

As you review the suggestions in Part II, it is important to remember that you can nourish your qi and increase the effectiveness of acupuncture by making smart dietary choices. The different elements of TCM are interdependent, just like the systems and parts of the human body, and they also affect your mood.

Mind-body connection. Where is this? Diseases of the soul are more dangerous and more numerous than those of the body.

—CICERO

CHAPTER 3

Yin and Yang Theory

Most people now recognize the yin/yang symbol. You may have seen it on bumper stickers, T-shirts, yoga clothes, or in martial arts studios. It represents the fine balance of yin and yang in our bodies, in nature, and in life. It's the balance of hot and cold, moist and dry, day and night, action and rest, aggression and passivity, male and female. Yin and yang exist in every organ and in all aspects of life: in people, in other animals, and in nature. The concept originally comes from Taoism, a religious belief system dating back to the third or fourth century BC in China. Everything yang has a little yin in it, and vice versa. Both yin and yang are a part of, and have an impact on, your physical health. Let me explain in further detail what yin and yang actually are.

Yin is the black parts of the circle. It represents nighttime, water, slow movements, contraction, dissension, below, the front of the body, internal, softness, the Earth, female energy, nourishment, blood, rest, moisture, and contemplation. It regulates female hormones. Yin in the body helps keep the body cool, especially in the evening. Without enough of it you can experience night sweats, which is the case for many menopausal women. Yin contributes to the making of blood. It is also calming, thus preventing anxiety.

Yang is the white of the circle. It represents daytime, light, sun, fire, above, expansion, the back of the body, the exterior, rapid movement, hardness, male energy, testosterone, action, and the heavens. It warms the body, promotes circulation of qi and blood, and provides energy. Yang helps to get you going in the morning or running in an emergency. Without enough of it, you may feel tired or cold much of the time.

Keeping yang and yin in harmony is a very delicate balance and necessary for optimal health. Without this harmony, illness, discomfort, and emotional issues will occur. Yin and yang cannot exist without each other. If yin starts to go out of balance, a yang imbalance will soon follow, and vice versa. If yin becomes weak or deficient, yang becomes excessive. Eventually the cycle turns, and the conditions become the opposite: yin excess, yang deficiency. Without lifestyle changes, herbs, and proper nutrition, the imbalance can go on indefinitely and become more and more severe, resulting in illness, mood swings, or serious health issues.

Catching a cold that turns into bronchitis is an example of the balance and interconnectedness of yin and yang. Someone who initially comes down with a cold might start off a little achy, with perhaps a slight increase in body temperature and a scratchy throat. If left untreated and without rest, the fever rises; maybe there will be alternate chills and fever. The fever becomes higher and higher, and sweating occurs. All symptoms will become worse. The scratchy throat becomes a severe sore throat; a cough with yellow or green phlegm develops. Eventually the high fever can turn into severe chills. No matter how many blankets you have to cover you, you're freezing. Eventually symptoms improve, with everything going in the reverse order from which it started. Severe chills, then a fever that goes down. Phlegm goes from green to yellow to white. Aches and coughing become less intense. Eventually you're back to normal. Yin and yang are balanced.

The main source of yin and yang is the kidneys. If the kidneys are weak, yin and/or yang will more than likely be insufficient for the entire body. They can be increased and nourished through proper treatment and lifestyle changes. Modern living weakens the kidneys. Excessive work, not enough sleep, stress, poor eating habits, medications, drugs, and alcohol—they all have an effect on the health of the kidneys and how much yin and yang they can make and store. As I've pointed out with other modern medical "discoveries," TCM was able to connect the dots centuries before anything else. Another prime example is that the adrenal glands, which are in charge of our response to stress, are considered one organ with the kidneys, and the kidneys in TCM are weakened by stress.

Not having enough yin or yang can manifest in so many ways. Here are a few examples.

Lungs. Smoking depletes the yin of the lungs, which can lead to a hacking, dry cough. A dry cough that just won't go away after you've had the flu can result from the depletion of yin in your lungs. Without enough yin in your lungs, you might have a hard time crying or processing grief.

Stomach. Have you ever been totally starving but couldn't think of what to eat? You stare into the fridge and nothing looks good, not even your favorite guacamole or coconut milk ice cream. This may indicate a lack of yin in your stomach. This may manifest as obsessive thinking, even to the point of obsessive-compulsive disorder.

Kidneys. Ah, the glories of menopause. Not every woman experiences the joys of night sweats and hot flashes, but those who do probably need to nourish the yin in their kidneys. Do you tend to feel cold and sense weak knees or low back pain? Feel anxious a lot? Then you probably need to nourish the yang of your kidneys.

Spleen. Hopefully, this has never happened to you, but some people experience diarrhea on a daily basis. TCM points not to an infection, food allergies, or a parasite, but to a deficiency of yang in the spleen. Being a worrywart or overthinker can also be a sign of a weak spleen.

Heart. Heart symptoms are most likely to show up as what we know as heart issues, such as heart disease, heart attacks, and irregular heartbeat. But this isn't always the case. Not enough yang in the heart can lead to palpitations, angina, and sadness from, for example, a relationship breakup that just won't lessen. Deficiency of yin in the heart can manifest as lupus, Types I and II diabetes, and hyperthyroidism.

Liver. The liver is charge of removing toxins from the body, and as such it is an organ that gets abused in the world we live into today. Most people have at least one symptom related to not enough yin in the liver, such as waking at 3 a.m.; dry nails, eyes, or throat; and constipation. Illnesses may include asthma, anemia, tremors, and liver cancer.

Stuart came to me with several yang deficiency symptoms. His chief complaint was low back pain. His lower back and glutes were cool to the touch. Stuart also felt cold unless it was over 80 degrees Fahrenheit; he just couldn't get warm. He also had low energy and very slow metabolism. Stuart started to feel better immediately after adding yang-boosting or warming foods and getting acupuncture to increase his yang. His energy levels increased, and his pain went away in just a couple of weeks.

Now you know what the yin/yang symbol means. Their balance is key to a balanced life. Yin and yang are an indispensable part of TCM, and you can use this new knowledge and the information in Parts II and III to help pick the right foods for whatever ails you.

The doctor of the future will give no medicine, but will interest her or his patients in the care of the human frame, in a proper diet, and in the cause and prevention of disease.

—THOMAS EDISON

CHAPTER 4

It's Elemental

The trees (or Wood), the sun (or Fire), the Earth, Metal, and Water. For the Chinese, these five elements are what make up all of existence. They play a role in nature and in our health. Without a sound balance of all five elements, each of them doing their part, and interacting and supporting each other, we cannot live a balanced life.

So what does this have to do with being happy?

Just as the yin and yang theory is an integral part of TCM, the 5-element theory is also very important in helping you decide which foods are best for your whole body health. Each of the elements—Wood, Fire, Earth, Metal, and Water—is related to specific organs, illnesses, and emotions. As with most Chinese medical theories, the 5-element theory is based on the natural cycles of nature and the body. Each of the five elements is closely related to pairs of organs, one organ being a yin organ, the other yang.

Each element is also connected to particular emotions—anger, heartbreak, worry, grief, and fear—as well as a specific season, tastes, colors, and even planets. The Earth element, for example, is paired with the spleen and the stomach, and related to overthinking, late summer, sweet tastes, the color yellow, and (not surprisingly) planet Earth. Much of the time, it is a good idea to eat foods that bear the same color as the color associated with the organ/element. Thus, a naturally occurring color like the yellow of squash is great for the Earth element, and the spleen and stomach. As you will learn, black is the key color for the Water element, so black beans nourish the kidneys and bladder and help fix Water imbalances, as well as address fear and anxiety.

What is meant by the taste of an element? If you have a weakness of a certain element/organ, you might crave certain tastes or flavors, and foods with this specific flavor will benefit or worsen your condition. The tastes associated with 5-element theory are sour, sweet, bitter, spicy, and salty. But remember that the sweetness found in most sugary items and the saltiness in processed foods are not beneficial. Sorry! Only naturally occurring flavors and tastes support wellness.

For example, when your Water element is weak or imbalanced, you may crave salty foods. You might suffer from anxiety and have low back pain or ringing in the ears. Salty foods (as long as it's not from excess or chemically processed salt, such as monosodium glutamate or refined table salt) will benefit your kidneys. But remember, bacon, pizza, and potato chips will impair your kidneys and bladder. Naturally salty sea vegetables, such as seaweed—nori and kelp—would be good for someone with a Water imbalance.

Once again, please keep in mind that saying an organ is imbalanced doesn't necessarily mean the actual organ. So don't worry if you have symptoms of a liver, or Wood, imbalance. An actual problem with the organ in question should only be determined by consulting your physician.

I'll be using the terms *manifests, benefits,* and *opens to* in relation to an organ and its associations with other parts of the body. What do I mean by this? When an organ or element is out of whack, it will present itself in ways we're not used to connecting in our Western mind-set. One example is that a heart imbalance can manifest on the tongue, which may cause speech issues like a lisp or an inability to get words out, or even muteness. You may also recognize this by a lack of joy in your life. A Wood imbalance may be noticeable by a presence of anger and can cause blurry vision or dry eyes, because the liver "opens to" the eyes in TCM.

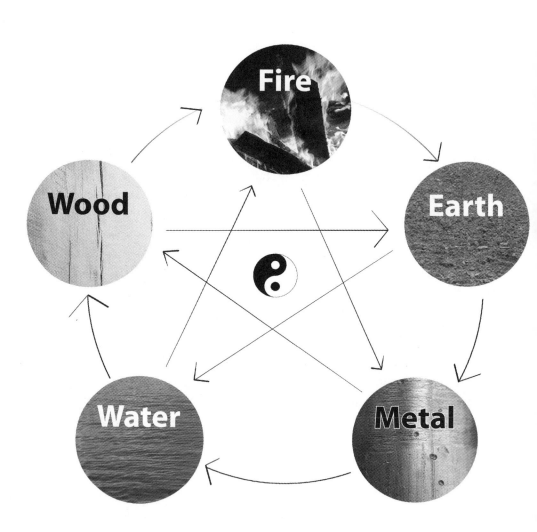

5 Elements

	WOOD	FIRE	EARTH	METAL	WATER
Viscera	Liver	Heart	Spleen	Lung	Kidney
Bowels	Gall Bladder	Small Intestine	Stomach	Large Intestine	Urinary Bladder
Five Sense Organs	Eye	Tongue	Mouth	Nose	Ear
Five Tissues	Tendon	Blood Vessel	Muscle	Skin & Hair	Bone
Emotions	Anger, Frustration, Resentment	Joy	Overthinking	Grief	Fear
Season	Spring	Summer	Late Summer	Autumn	Winter
Environment	Wind	Heat	Dampness	Dryness	Cold
Sound	Calling Sound	Laughing	Singing	Crying	Deep Sighing
Color	Green	Red	Yellow	White	Black
Taste	Sour	Bitter	Sweet	Spicy	Salty
Direction	East	South	Middle	West	North
Time of Day	11 p.m. - 3 a.m.	11 a.m. - 3 p.m.	7 a.m. - 11 a.m.	3 a.m. - 7 a.m.	3 p.m. - 7 p.m.

The chart on p. 23 gives a quick overview of what each element represents. Let's delve in deeper and see what they're all about.

WOOD

Let's start with the Wood element, which is related to the liver (yin) and gallbladder (yang). Wood is associated with spring; it is a time for rebirth. This is easy to remember: Think about trees and their growth during this time. People who have a weak Wood element tend to have their symptoms aggravated or get sick more often at this time of year. The taste associated with Wood is sour, and the color is green. The main emotions associated with Wood are anger, frustration, and resentment. Dark, leafy greens such as kale, broccoli, and spinach support the Wood element and can help balance these emotions. This is another example of how ahead of its time Chinese nutrition has always been, especially when compared with Western nutrition, which now accepts that dark greens support the liver and help flush out toxins.

Case Study: Steven was an active alcoholic looking for help in getting sober. He had recently been diagnosed with cirrhosis of the liver after blood found in his stools sent him to the hospital for tests. While Steven would drink a fifth of vodka before going to work every morning, he definitely wasn't your stereotypical drunk. He was the CEO of a major corporation, divorced with one child, and worked out six days a week. Steven was known for his fits of rage, but somehow this didn't keep him from being highly respected in his field. He came in to see me also complaining of high blood pressure and cholesterol, fatigue, yellowing of the skin, and occasional disorientation, which he attributed to intoxication. While his alcoholism was a cause, from the perspective of TCM, he suffered from an imbalance in the Wood element. My first food suggestion for Steven was to drink a green juice three times a day to aid in his detoxification and support his liver. His green juice consisted of celery, spinach, kale, romaine lettuce, cucumber, an apple, cilantro, parsley, and ginger. Steven kept to his sobriety and now lives free from the anger he used to spew out onto everyone around him.

FIRE

The heart and small intestines are the yin and yang organs, respectively, of Fire. Summer is the season of Fire, which is easy to remember since it's the hottest time of year. It is a time for growth, and those with a weak Fire element will have their symptoms worsen during the summer months. The associated taste is bitter, and the color is red. Heartache and lack of joy affect the Fire element. Red fruits like strawberries and pomegranates nourish the heart and work to appease these emotions.

Case Study: After the death of his wife of forty-five years, Benjamin's heart was broken into a million pieces. Benjamin said he experienced chest pain constantly, but his doctors said his heart was fine. He was a very stoic, old-fashioned guy who didn't like to share or express his feelings with anyone. But Benjamin was so distraught over the loss of his wife that he opened up to me. I recommended he eat beets, radish, red bell peppers, and saffron, all foods designed to nourish his heart. Benjamin slowly started to heal and eventually met a girlfriend he adored.

EARTH

The organs associated with the Earth element are the spleen (yin) and stomach (yang). Earth's season is late summer, notably the transition of summer to fall, the time of harvest. People with a weak Earth element will experience more symptoms during this time of year. Worry, overthinking, and obsessive thoughts can weaken the Earth element. The Earth element has a corresponding color of yellow and is sweet in taste. Mangoes, oranges, and peanuts all support and strengthen this element.

Case Study: Sugar addicts all have weakened spleens. Did the weak spleen come first, causing the cravings? Or did overindulging in sugar cause a weak spleen? It's hard to say for sure. Sally drank two liters of soda every day and usually enjoyed a dessert with lunch and dinner. She was a Type II diabetic and diagnosed with obsessive-compulsive disorder (OCD). Sally literally couldn't stop worrying. She spent hours every day concerned about germs and whether her home was locked. Sally was even thinking of quitting her job to avoid getting sick and to make sure her house was safe. It's no wonder she had a sickly spleen. Getting Sally off sugar took a while, but once she quit, her OCD symptoms lessened.

METAL

The element of Metal is also paired with two organs, the lungs holding the yin, and large intestines holding the yang. Metal is connected to fall, the time of transformation and shedding old habits. The affiliated taste is pungent or spicy; the color is white. People with a weak Metal element are prone to being sick during the fall. Grief and sadness can also cause an imbalance in the lungs and large intestine. Pears are a healthy and delicious way of healing the Metal element.

Case Study: Laurence was the prime example of someone whose cravings were the result of his health problems. He loved spicy food. He would put hot sauce, peppers, or cayenne pepper on everything—even foods you wouldn't think to make spicy, like tuna salad or macaroni and cheese. He bought jalapeños like there would soon be a shortage. Laurence also had several health issues that made sense when viewed as an imbalance in his Metal element. He had suffered from asthma and eczema since he was a toddler. He had bronchitis every November for as long as he could remember. Laurence also suffered from irritable bowel syndrome (IBS), with abdominal cramping and painful diarrhea daily. He knew the spicy foods were probably aggravating his IBS, but he couldn't help himself. After about a month of treatments Laurence shared that he never resolved the death of his father when he was six years old. He knew logically that it was OK to move on, but he just couldn't. With all of his lung and large intestine concerns, it was no wonder he loved his peppers. I suggested he eat sweet potatoes, kale, spinach, tofu, cabbage, miso soup, and oranges regularly. As he got healthier, the need to continually burn his mouth lessened.

WATER

In TCM terms, this element is related to the kidneys and the bladder, which are the yin and yang organs of Water. The color of the Water element is black, and its taste is salty. It correlates to winter—the time to go inside, rest, and get ready for rebirth in spring. Fear and anxiety are the main emotions related to the kidneys and bladder, which can be helped by eating black foods such as wild rice and black sesame seeds.

Case Study: Anxiety is one of the more common concerns I see in my clinic. Helen was diagnosed with post-traumatic stress disorder and anxiety after serving in Iraq, where she'd seen things no one should have to see. Her anxiety made it almost impossible for her to function normally. She also ate salty, fried foods at every meal. Hash browns, french fries, potato chips, mozzarella sticks, and lots of Chinese food were her staples, which falls right in line with how TCM looks at food cravings relating to specific organs and emotions. Helen's Water element was so weak from her experience as a soldier that she wanted salt all the time, which harmed her health. Over-consumption of white table salt and monosodium glutamate was making her Water element weaker and the cravings even stronger. She should eat only naturally occurring salty foods such as seaweed, celery, or artichoke. After I explained to Helen why she craved all this salt, she switched to seaweed snacks and celery sticks to satisfy her salt cravings, and we got her anxiety a little bit under control.

The basic information in this chapter should help you understand the 5-element theory and its relation to Chinese nutrition. As you can now also see, nature is a reflection of our bodies and vice versa. Finding the right things to eat for what ails you is as simple as counting to five.

All that man needs for health and healing has been provided by God in nature, the Challenge of science is to find it.

— PHILIPPUS AUREOLUS THEOPHRASTUS BOMBAST VON HOHENHEIM, KNOWN AS PARACELSUS (1493–1541)

CHAPTER 5

Herbalicious

No, I don't mean *those* kinds of herbs. And, yes, I do get asked that—a lot.

The healing properties of herbs were discovered through trial and error, and also during the observation of animals. Animals instinctively know what to eat to help them. Early herbologists began their studies by observing animals eating specific plants and achieving very specific results. For example, when animals were seen eating the root of ginseng, there were subsequent signs of an increase in energy.

I also see this natural instinct and response in the small children I treat. One of my autistic patients, age five, would grab her bottle of powdered herbs out of her parents' hands. Sylvia was severely autistic when she first came to see me. She only spoke to mimic what someone else said, was unable to feed herself, couldn't make eye contact at all, would only wear certain colors, ate just about ten foods of a particular texture, had issues with anger and temper tantrums, and still wasn't potty trained. But she knew her herbs were making her feel better. She lit up when she took them, three times a day—and for any of you who have taken Chinese herbs, fresh or in powder, you know how awful they can taste! Yet almost all my younger pediatric patients (five and under) have the same response as Sylvia. They intuitively know the herbs are helping and don't care or don't even notice the taste. Very small children have to use liquid or powdered herbs until they are able to swallow capsules, but remarkable results are possible.

Sylvia's results were nothing short of miraculous. She was seeing several other health-care providers and specialists beside me, so I can't take all the credit, but her parents did comment that after her sessions with me, the response was always quite drastic. Once Sylvia was feeling much better, she eventually changed her diet as well. If you've been around a child with autism, you know that you can't make them do anything they don't want to; dietary changes came after about a month of treatments. Sylvia was able to make eye contact, albeit for only a few seconds, after just three weeks. Her tantrums, which used to last hours, were practically gone right away. Within a year, her autism spectrum symptoms were essentially gone, noticeable only in situations when she felt shy or didn't understand social cues.

Chinese herbs are another incredibly powerful healing modality in TCM. Acupuncture and proper nutrition can do wonders in healing, even for conditions that many think are "unhealable." Adding a special herbal formula to the treatment can vastly improve any emotional and physical issues and quicken recovery time drastically.

Chinese herbs are very complex and should be studied thoroughly before prescribing. This is why I highly recommend only going to a qualified licensed practitioner for herbal remedies. Each state has its own laws about prescribing Chinese herbs. In California, where I'm licensed, I had to study herbs along with acupuncture to qualify for a license. About one-fifth of my class hours were spent learning Chinese herbology as part of my curriculum. I had to memorize the healing properties and contraindications of hundreds of Chinese herbs to graduate. In California, 11 percent of the state board exam is on herbs.

Chinese herbology is a science and an art form. Each herb has its own healing properties. Some have several. Each herb has a recommended dose to it. For example, the dose for ginseng is from 1 gram to 9 grams, depending on your condition and what other herbs you are combining with it. If you've experienced severe blood loss from an injury or childbirth, the dose goes up to 30 grams. How much you use determines how effective it is and its purpose. How an herb is prepared also changes its healing capabilities. Whether it's prepared fried, raw, dried, or freeze-dried can all tweak an herb's effects. Also, each part of a plant has very specific properties and uses. The bark might not have the same effect as the leaf, root, seed, or berry. For example, most people have heard gingko biloba helps with memory. Yes, it does—at least the seeds do—but in TCM the *leaf* is used for asthma, chest colds, and other lung-related illnesses.

PATENT FORMULAS

There are herbal remedies that are called patent formulas. They're premade concoctions that address a specific ailment, sometimes even a few. You might even be able to buy some of them at your local health food store. For example, there are traditional formulas that treat sinus infections, bladder infections, muscle aches and injuries, anxiety, and digestive problems. These offer an excellent way to focus on and treat a specific and acute condition. Patent formulas can also be used for more chronic conditions, such as hay fever or long-term insomnia.

I prefer starting my new patients with one of these formulas. I see how they're doing for a few weeks, make sure they're consistently taking their herbs, then I make a specialized formula that treats many, if not all, of their problems. I make sure they're consistently taking their supplements, because many people just aren't wired to do that. I can't tell you how many patients come in with grocery bags of vitamins and herbal supplements they've had sometimes for years. They have no idea why they bought most of them, and a majority of the bottles are expired. We end up throwing away sometimes hundreds of dollars of unusable or unnecessary products. You *can* get some benefit by occasionally taking herbs or vitamins, just as you reap *some* rewards from occasionally eating fruits and vegetables. But the best results come from consistency, to give you a cumulative effect. I don't want people to spend money on supplements that are just going to sit in their medicine cabinets and be forgotten. I also prescribe premade herbal formulas when a patient comes in with a new symptom, like a chest cold or stomach flu. Taking herbs this way can knock out a bug pretty quickly, so something that would normally last days or even weeks can be gone in just a few days.

At least one patient a day comes into my clinic with a cold or flu. So I keep plenty of cold-busting formulas on hand. My immediate goals are to relieve symptoms and get rid of the infection by boosting the immune system. There's no need to be coughing out a lung for weeks on end! Once the cold symptoms are gone, I give herbs that will prevent future infection. Herbs can take care of it all.

Then there are custom-made herbal formulas. I'd say about 80 percent of my patients take a special formula. These are a mix of several different Chinese herbs that are specific to each patient. I take into consideration each herb I use in a formula, because they can have a synergistic effect with other herbs in a formula, increasing or decreasing its effectiveness. Chinese herbs work in harmony and can have better results, depending on the combination and dosage. For example, if constipation is your chief complaint, but you also suffer from headaches and premenstrual syndrome (PMS), your special formula will contain herbs that treat each of these problems. The focus is on constipation, but the formula will also reduce or eliminate your headaches and PMS. This way your practitioner works on several issues without prescribing several different pills. I can tell you from clinical and personal experience that Chinese herbs can eradicate or at least drastically reduce the symptoms of most illnesses, even those considered incurable by Western medicine.

Herbs can also be helpful in treating infertility, an issue for almost seven million American women between the ages of fifteen and forty-four. Patty was thirty-six when she first came to see me. She had been trying to get pregnant for four years with no luck. Patty, unfortunately, had two early-term miscarriages during that time. She tried every type of Western treatment imaginable, including nine attempts with in vitro fertilization. Yes, nine times. Her periods were always regular, and her hormone levels were considered in the normal range. Patty's doctors had given up, and Patty was about to give up as well. Luckily, one of her coworkers whom I had helped with similar problems suggested coming to me. After just three months of herbs, acupuncture, and some simple dietary changes, Patty became pregnant. She now has a healthy six-year-old boy.

Fertility is one gynecological issue where TCM takes a very different approach than Western medicine. It's important that a patient's hormones be at the appropriate levels to conceive, of course, but in TCM fertility is much more than a bunch of numbers. I can only speak from my own clinical experience on this, but I've helped at least eighty couples conceive that were considered lost causes, just like Patty. There is almost always an emotional component to infertility that also needs to be dealt with, along with an energetic component. Many of my female patients with gynecological issues, such as infertility, endometriosis, severe cramps, and fibroids, have an energetic blockage "down there."

Chinese herbs can heal fertility issues in men as well. Men usually respond very quickly to the protocol I give them. Whether it's low sperm count, low motility, oddly shaped sperm, impotence, low libido, or weak sperm, Chinese herbs are very powerful in improving male fertility without medications or hormones. Dave and his wife were trying to conceive for almost a year before he got his sperm tested. All his numbers were very poor. Dave was retested after just seven weeks of Chinese herbs and everything had improved. As an added bonus, he had a lot more energy, and his short temper was practically gone. Three months later Dave's wife was pregnant.

Reproductive organs of men and women are related to the liver channel. This is because liver channel wraps around the genitals. So whenever there's a blockage in the uterus or testes, I treat the liver channel with herbs and acupuncture. Herbs are the perfect way to remove any accumulations or excesses in the reproductive organs. Many women with fertility concerns have experienced some type of sexual trauma. It doesn't have to be as traumatic as rape—it can be sexual harassment, feeling unsafe or upset in a sexual situation, or being ogled by a neighbor while growing up. I can't say this is the case with every woman dealing with fertility, but it's very common. Once the incident or incidents have been processed and released, most women get pregnant pretty quickly.

Many people hear about the "weird" stuff that can be used in Chinese herbal medicine, such as deer antler, bugs, and the like. I personally only use plant sources, such as berries, leaves, roots, flowers, and bark, for all my formulas. This isn't just because of my own lifestyle. Most Western folks are uncomfortable with the idea of drinking a tea with cicada shells in it. If you're at all concerned about this in regard to your own herbalist, make sure to bring it up. Most Western-trained acupuncturists know to mention what's in a formula to their patients, but not all actually do it. Also, please note that things like bear bile are illegal to use anyway!

If taken correctly, Chinese herbs have no negative side effects. Unfortunately, people sometimes take them in extremely high doses (five to ten times the recommended dose or more) and can get very sick. Usually, this overdosing is done for weight loss. So when you hear of a completely safe and commonly used Chinese herb being taken off the market due to safety, it's because people abused it. Herbs are very powerful, just like drugs, so taking them properly is important. Consulting with a licensed professional is always a good idea when taking herbal supplements, not just for safety, but also to guarantee you get the best results possible.

Chinese herbs are usually taken two or three times a day. Sometimes they can be taken less, such as once before bed to combat insomnia, or more often, such as every few hours to combat an acute condition, such as a sinus infection. But in general, taking Chinese herbs two or three times a day is all that's necessary to benefit from them. You're probably used to taking Western medication once or possibly twice a day. Chinese herbs—at least how I prescribe them—haven't been chemically altered to fit in one tiny pill. Keeping herbs as close to their natural state as possible guarantees their efficacy.

There can be some crossover between Western and Chinese herbs. I get asked all the time what I think of a particular Western herb, such as ginseng and gingko biloba, as mentioned earlier. Many Americans have heard of, and even tried, ginseng and licorice root, which have been used in China for centuries. Sometimes I know about it because it's also in the Chinese herbal pharmacy or I've done research. I don't like to give an opinion unless I know the herb or supplement well.

Ginseng

I'll use the example of ginseng to help you see how Chinese herbs work and how specific herbal medicine is. First, it's important to know there are different types of ginseng: Korean, Chinese, American, and Siberian. Each kind has its own set of healing properties, but some of them overlap. Because the plant's root often grows to resemble a human body, the name *ginseng* is a combination of the Chinese words for "man" and "plant." All the names of herbs and acupoints have a meaning, which stems from the history of how people learned what the herbs did, how they looked, possibly where to find them, and sometimes their spiritual significance.

All the different types of ginseng boost the immune system to prevent illness; reduce stress, anger, and frustration; aid in liver function; improve digestion; increase libido and sexual stamina; and enhance energy levels. In addition, American ginseng reduces or cures menopausal disorders and reduces fever and cough. Siberian ginseng improves memory. Korean ginseng prevents cancer, helps with diabetes, and aids in mental focus.

And something I probably shouldn't be telling you . . . ginseng reduces the effects of alcohol and alleviates hangovers.

Ginseng is one of those wonder herbs that can do so much. The older it is, the stronger it gets. You can make a tea out of the root, cook it in soup, or stir-fry it with your favorite veggies and tempeh. But remember that ginseng is not recommended if you are already suffering from a cold or the flu, as it can actually nourish an infection instead getting rid of it.

Ginger

Another Chinese herb that you might already have in your spice rack is ginger. Ginger has many more functions than just tasting great or helping with an upset tummy (in the form of ginger ale). Sushi lovers will be glad to know why it's almost always served with raw fish: Ginger kills parasites, warms the belly, and aids in the digestion of fatty foods. Ginger is also an immune booster. So, if you're fighting the flu or have been around sick people at work, have some ginger tea, juice it, or eat it in your carrot soup. It has very strong anti-inflammatory properties to reduce pain and swelling. Ginger also thins the blood to prevent heart attacks and stroke. It aids in the release of toxins by strengthening the kidneys and stimulating perspiration. If you suffer from cold hands and feet, it also helps with circulation. Ginger minimizes worry. You can eat it, drink it, or even add some to your bath. This little root can heal almost anything and should be called a panacea.

John came in complaining of food poisoning. He was exposed to salmonella in his morning scrambled eggs almost two weeks before coming in for treatment. He still felt nauseated most of the time, had no appetite, was very weak, and had diarrhea at least three times a day. Poor John was miserable. I gave him ginger tea before starting his treatment, and an herbal formula, which included dried ginger, to take four times a day until his symptoms improved. John e-mailed me the next afternoon with the great news that he was already better.

Turmeric

Turmeric, the herb that makes curry yellow and gives it that extra zing, is a powerhouse of healing properties. In Chinese medicine this little yellow root is mostly used for inflammation and, even more specifically, for shoulder pain. But there are many other health benefits of turmeric: It has been recommended for the treatment of skin conditions, reducing pain, improving metabolism, detoxifying blood, diminishing overthinking and obsessive thoughts, reducing gas and bloating, accelerating wound healing, moderating the effects of asthma, lowering cholesterol, healing stomach ulcers, slowing the progression of multiple sclerosis and Alzheimer's disease, and reducing the side effects of chemotherapy—and the list goes on from there.

As with all herbs, fresh is always best, but powdered and capsule forms will still help quite a bit. Turmeric can be added to soups, stews, grilled veggies, tofu scramble, and, of course, curry. Juice a small amount with some cucumber, carrots, lemon, and lettuce for a delicious, immune-boosting treat every morning. You can also make it into a paste with aloe vera to reduce itching from bug bites and chicken pox.

Cinnamon

Then there's cinnamon. I grew up having cinnamon on applesauce. But my favorite way to eat it was on toasted Wonder bread with butter and sugar as a sweet dinner treat. Totally healthy, right? Well, at least there was cinnamon on there.

It's not just delicious; it's really good for you. Cinnamon has many healing properties and tastes great with all root veggies and fruits (and white bread). It is high in fiber, manganese, iron, and calcium. It helps regulate blood sugar, improves memory, removes toxins from the blood, and aids circulation because it includes a blood-thinning compound. It has antifungal, antibacterial, antiviral, and antiseptic properties. Because of its anti-inflammatory and circulation properties, cinnamon helps reduce pain, stiffness, and menstrual cramps. It helps with indigestion, releasing grief, morning sickness, nausea, vomiting, diarrhea, and flatulence. It also helps combat the symptoms of colds and the flu, such as sore throat and congestion. It even increases the secretion of breast milk and freshens your breath.

Isn't it amazing how the things we have in our kitchen cabinet can keep us healthy? Every time we cook, we have the opportunity to improve our quality of life. As Hippocrates pointed out, food can really be thy medicine.

Health is a state of complete harmony of the body, mind, and spirit. When one is free from physical disabilities and mental distractions, the gates of the soul open.

—B. K. S. IYENGAR

CHAPTER 6

Diagnosis and Treatment with TCM

Before choosing the right herbs and foods for my patients, I first have to make a diagnosis and treatment plan. Chinese medicine has a unique way of diagnosing a patient. People who are new to acupuncture are amazed both by all the questions I ask and my examination: looking at the tongue, feeling the pulse for several minutes on both wrists, and palpating certain areas of the body. An initial intake can take up to an hour, depending on a patient's overall condition and history. During an initial visit I ask quite a few questions about medical history, supplements and medications, lifestyle choices, eating and exercise habits, and much more. I check the texture and temperature of the client's skin along certain energy channels; look at the complexion, hair quality, eyes, body type, and body language; and listen to the sound of the patient's voice. I sometimes even smell the patient. If I sense that a patient is open or ready to be asked, I'll ask about his or her emotional health and history as well. All of these help me in my diagnosis and to decide the best course of treatment for that particular individual.

Throughout this book, I'll be using some potentially unfamiliar terms when discussing my patients' symptoms. I want to make sure you have some background on how a diagnosis is made and how I decide on the best treatment for each of my patients. Do keep in mind that entire books have been written on each individual treatment method, so it would be impossible to summarize them all in only a few pages. Instead, I've taken some of the most vital information and simplified it. I am sharing some diagnostic tools with you here so you can see how exact TCM can be. Just remember that even if you see parallels with your own symptoms, please don't use this chapter to self-diagnose or to start taking herbs without the help of a qualified practitioner. What makes Chinese medicine so different from Western medicine is that each patient is looked at as a whole system, not just as a symptom or two. Every person is unique, with a unique life experience and set of symptoms and ways of processing his or her emotions. So finding out as much as I can about my patients is important to giving them the best possible treatment, diet suggestions and results. We will start with what can easily be seen in a preliminary interview.

FACE

You can tell a lot about the health of your organs and emotional health just by looking in the mirror. In TCM, it is believed that each organ and its correlating emotions manifest on a specific part of the face, so that a person's complexion may reflect his or her state of mind. Have you ever paid attention to the face of a person who yells to himself or herself? Next time, take a look at their face (without staring!) and see what it is telling you.

- The forehead represents the heart.
- The tip of the nose is the spleen.
- The chin is the kidneys.
- The liver is the left cheek.
- The lungs are reflected on the right cheek.

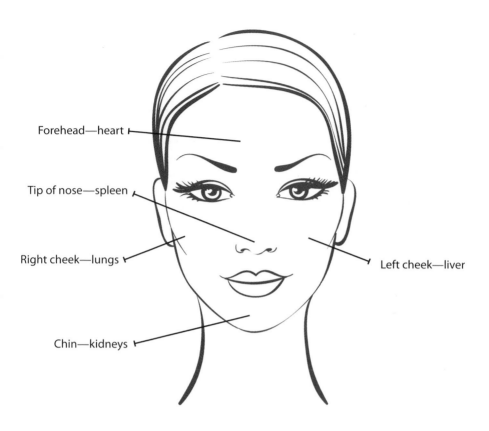

Forehead—heart

Tip of nose—spleen

Right cheek—lungs

Left cheek—liver

Chin—kidneys

Facial acne is one of most obvious ways to help diagnose a patient. Patients who always get acne on their cheeks may have imbalances in either their liver or lungs. Usually acne, especially in adults, is an indicator that the liver is trying to flush out toxins through the skin. The solution? Eat some more of those dark, leafy greens and ginger I mentioned earlier for a mini detox.

Having digestive issues may result in a red-tipped nose, which indicates a weak spleen. Sally, the sugar addict mentioned in chapter 4, had a bright red nose.

Specific colors can also be an indicator that something is wrong with a particular organ. These colors can show up on the face, in the eyes, or on the skin anywhere on the body. A green hue to the complexion can mean there is a liver issue, such as cirrhosis. Redness usually means some form of internal heat, such as a fever, infection, or menopause. Yellow can be a sign of digestive issues, such as

Acne

Isn't acne supposed to be a teenager's problem? You would think so. But people of all ages get acne, and for many reasons. Acne is a sign that your body needs some extra attention. It's an indication that something is off balance internally.

The causes of acne include the following:

- **Hormonal imbalances.** There are many causes of hormonal imbalances, including birth control pills, plastics, pesticides, and steroids.

- **Liver toxicity.** Adult-onset acne, especially cystic acne, can be a sign of toxin buildup in your liver.

- **Bacterial, fungal, or yeast overgrowth.** Your body tries flushing this overgrowth out through the skin.

- **Food allergies.** Acne is one of the many ways food allergies can manifest.

There are some really simple ways to eliminate or at least reduce acne. First, give up dairy for a week and see if your skin improves. It's one of the major causes of acne. Then avoid known food allergens and hormone-altering beauty products, cleaning products, and foods. Cleansers in your shower or under the kitchen sink may be the cause of your acne or other skin issues.

I also recommend doing a safe liver cleanse at least once a year. If you have pimples as an adult, this is a must. Your skin should start to clear up after flushing out toxins from your liver. I have my favorite liver cleanse products, but it's best to consult a qualified physician to choose the best products for you. A simple way you can purge the junk in your body on your own is to eat only raw fruits and veggies for a week. Make sure to eat lots of dark, leafy greens such as kale, dandelion greens, watercress, cilantro, and arugula. Drink only lemon water, fresh juices (especially from the dark, leafy greens above), and smoothies. During this week, take vitamin C, selenium, vitamin E, milk thistle, and chlorella to further support the liver in flushing out any noxious substances such as medications, chlorine from water, and heavy metals like mercury and lead.

indigestion, diarrhea, or stomach flu. A very pale complexion can mean you are anemic. Anemia may be caused by either lack of or malabsorption of iron and/or vitamin B_{12}.

EYES

Just like the skin of the face, the eyes can give you an idea of any imbalances in specific organs or their emotions. They're not just the windows to the soul. The eyes can tell what's going on internally.

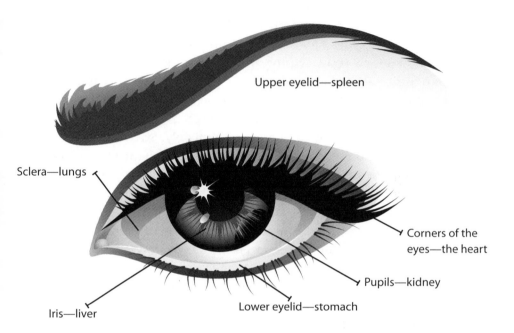

Upper eyelid—spleen

Sclera—lungs

Corners of the eyes—the heart

Pupils—kidney

Iris—liver

Lower eyelid—stomach

Dark circles under the eyes can signify kidney imbalance, food allergies, possible caffeine poisoning (too much coffee) of the kidneys, and/or adrenal fatigue.

If the eyes are dull and/or clouded, it may be an indication of serious mental health issues such as bipolar disorder. Dullness can also sometimes be a side effect of certain medications.

If the corners of the eyes are red, you may be experiencing anxiety or insomnia.

SWEAT

I see a lot of people who have issues with sweat. They might think their sweating is normal, because they've "always been this way," but it can be a sign that something is off balance internally. Like many symptoms, just because you've had the issue for years doesn't mean it's OK.

Sweating is a normal bodily function to regulate body temperature, but some types of sweating are abnormal. Anxiety especially affects how much you perspire, but any emotional imbalance can have an impact. You might sweat only on the head, which can mean, for example, heat in the stomach, stomach flu, or food poisoning, while sweat showing up solely on the forehead can mean a heart attack—and a need to see a doctor immediately. Sweat only on the arms and legs can mean a stomach or spleen deficiency and can be evidence of stress-induced digestion problems, eating disorders, or overuse of antibiotics. Sweat only on the hands can mean a lung qi deficiency or nerves, which can manifest as shortness of breath or frequent colds. If you sweat only during the day, it could mean a yang or qi deficiency, commonly seen in patients who always feel cold or tired. Sweat on the palms, soles of the feet, or chest can mean a yin deficiency, sometimes caused by menopause or cancer treatments. Finding emotional balance through increasing the right mood foods for you should stabilize your perspiration.

HEADACHES

Headaches are definitely a manifestation of imbalances. Unfortunately, they've become part of the norm. Common causes are eye strain from sitting in front of a computer too much and the overconsumption of caffeinated drinks, leading to dehydration. Depending on where on the head the pain is centered, or the quality of the pain itself, you can find out what organ(s) may need some TLC.

Headaches that occur only during the day may mean a qi or yang deficiency, which can manifest as fatigue or muscle weakness. By contrast, nighttime headaches can mean a blood or yin deficiency caused by anemia or the side effects of medications. Pain at the nape of the neck can mean a kidney deficiency, tight neck muscles, or

Cancer Treatments and TCM

Nobody wants to hear the C word. Unfortunately, we all know at least one person with cancer. One in three women and one in two men will have cancer in their lifetimes. Those are some scary statistics. But cancer doesn't have to be a death sentence. It can be a turning point to a new and improved you. I like to have my patients try to look at a cancer diagnosis as an opportunity to take charge of their health. Beating cancer can be done.

If you've opted for Western treatment, the side effects can be worse than the cancer symptoms. So why not be proactive and reduce symptoms and reduce the chance of reoccurrence?

In TCM, cancer treatment mostly affects the kidneys, liver, and lungs. Side effects from cancer treatment include hot flashes, nausea, vomiting, diarrhea, sweating, insomnia, fatigue, low immunity, liver toxicity, anxiety/stress, and skin burns. To balance these side effects, you'll want to consume foods that support and nourish those organs.

What you eat, herbal and vitamin supplements, stress reduction, and acupuncture can all help your recovery and prevent reoccurrence. Those wonder foods, ginger and turmeric, that you learned about in chapter 5, not only help with nausea and reduce inflammation but also boost the immune system.

Some oncologists are big fans of TCM, while others are concerned about drug and herb interactions. Believe me, there are plenty of herbs that are safe and can even improve Western cancer treatment. If you are concerned about taking herbs, then at least start with dietary changes. You can always take herbs when you're done with your Western treatment.

the onset of a cold. Aching temples could mean liver or gallbladder imbalances, or a cold or flu. Pain at the vertex (top of the skull) is usually a sign of anemia. For example, my patient John with food poisoning had been complaining of a constant headache on the top of his head ever since getting sick. Because he was unable to keep anything down, he was dehydrated and anemic. Once he was able to eat and drink normally again, the headache disappeared. Pretty amazing, right? As I wrote earlier, these are just a few of many examples of the diagnostic tools used in TCM. But they should give you an idea of how many factors are taken into account when treating patients with this approach.

As you can now see, TCM isn't really that weird. It makes perfect sense. The masters from thousands of years ago had it right. Treating the cause of illness using natural methods provides for a long, healthy, disease-free life.

PART II

Emotional Rescue . . .
with Food

If you are patient in one moment of anger, you will escape a hundred days of sorrow.

—CHINESE PROVERB

CHAPTER 7

Angry Much?

ANGER

Recommended Foods

For anger in general, eat lima beans, raspberries, celery, and leeks.

If you experience any PMS symptoms or flank (sides of torso) pain, are holding on to resentment and anger, or are easily angered, the qi in your liver is probably stagnant. This means qi isn't flowing properly in your liver, leading to the above symptoms. You should eat plenty of these foods: beets, mustard greens, turnips, cabbage, cauliflower, broccoli, quinoa, asparagus, rye, romaine lettuce, alfalfa, pine nuts, brussels sprouts, vinegars (brown rice, rice wine, and apple cider), spices (dill, cumin, fennel, black pepper, marjoram, ginger, cardamom, onion, basil, mint, turmeric, bay leaf, and horseradish), and fruit (strawberries, peaches, and cherries).

When you've been exposed to any toxins, you definitely want to eat these foods on a regular, if not daily, basis: cucumber, mung beans, tofu, millet, plums, radish, rhubarb, daikon radish, spirulina, lettuce, kelp, nori, kombu, wakame, chlorella, parsley, kale, collard greens, and sprouts (alfalfa, sunflower, clover, mung, broccoli, and bean). Unfortunately, the world we live in is full of toxins. Our food, water, air, even clothing and beauty products, can contain harmful chemicals. So I recommend eating from this list every day.

When you experience menopause, hot flashes, night sweats, insomnia, hot hands and feet, dry mouth, and/or any chemotherapy side effects, there are plenty of tasty foods that reduce your symptoms. As all of these symptoms are the result of too little yin in your liver, you can benefit from these **yin-nourishing foods:** parsley, artichoke, carrots, avocado, lemon, lime, mulberries, yams, parsnips, oils (hemp, black currant, and flaxseed), and aloe vera gel.

Liver blood deficiency basically means you're anemic. Note that this might not even show up on a blood test. Symptoms of anemia include light-headedness, muscle cramps, leg cramps, fatigue, pale nail bed, shortness of breath, and poor concentration. Here are some goodies to build your blood: blackstrap molasses, soybeans, lentils, spinach, collard greens, blackberries, raspberries, prunes, and grapes.

Neurological issues can be the result of an unhappy liver in TCM. It's called "liver wind" when you have any of these health concerns: Parkinson's, multiple sclerosis, epilepsy, tremors, stroke, and seizures. You can calm the "wind" with these tasty treats: celery, oats, flaxseeds, black soybeans, pine nuts, black sesame seeds, basil, sage, fennel, anise, peppermint, chamomile, coconut, ginger, and strawberries.

Foods to Avoid or Minimize

For liver qi stagnation: spicy food

For liver wind: white flour, white rice, animal fats, and processed foods

For liver toxicity: sugar, alcohol, coffee, processed food, food coloring, food additives, and pesticides

Have you paid attention to what makes you angry? Do you let it out in the moment? Ignore it? Save expressing it for later once you've had a chance to process it? Do you have rage that seems to come from nowhere?

Anger is that emotion we all want to ignore. It can come out in unexpected bursts or, more predictably, when someone we love pushes our buttons. Sometimes you can experience an intense rush when feeling angry, but there's usually an emotional or physical crash afterward.

Expressing your anger in public is considered taboo. Women especially aren't supposed to get angry. We're considered bitchy or worse if we allow ourselves to get pissed off. Followers of TCM believe that this suppression of anger makes PMS much worse for many women.

So even if you're great at feeling your feelings, you probably suppress anger on a somewhat regular basis. Anger begins to build up in our livers, causing qi there to stagnate, and it can feel like a pressure cooker. That's why just screaming it out or punching someone in a kickboxing class feels so damn good.

As you learned in chapter 4, the Wood element is associated with the liver (yin) and gallbladder (yang), springtime, and anger. In TCM, the Wood element is linked to growth, the eyes, and nourishing the muscles and nails, so anything health-related in regard to muscles, nails, or eyes means the liver needs to be treated. I'll be giving a detailed list of symptoms associated with the liver and gallbladder later in the chapter, but just to give you an idea, if you're suffering from muscle tension and have brittle nails, most likely there's an imbalance in your liver.

As you learned earlier, each organ has its own set of emotions connected to it. These unexpressed but all-too-often experienced emotions can cause an imbalance in the organ. Or the imbalanced organ can lead you to feel these emotions more often, or amplified beyond normal levels. It can turn into the vicious cycle I discussed in chapter 1. This means that when you experience a certain emotion such as anger—and especially if you stuff down that anger—your liver will become compromised in some way. The reverse is also true: If the liver isn't working properly, you may experience outbursts of anger or make impulsive decisions.

Out of all the organs, the liver has the most emotions attached to it.

The emotions most directly affecting the liver are:

- **anger**
- **frustration**
- **hate**
- **rage**
- **resentment**

The liver is also a factor in:

- **control issues**
- **edginess**
- **moodiness**
- **being too impulsive or too rigid**
- **inability to keep commitments**
- **instability**
- **manic depression**
- **indecisiveness**

Any of these sound familiar?

A person with a healthy Wood element will be very balanced. They are able to forgive, make decisions easily, are reliable and confident, have hope and a vision for what the future holds, and are even tempered. Balanced Woods will be flexible but still stand strong in who they are and what they want. Imagine a tree. For it to grow and be indestructible, a tree has to have strong roots, a strong foundation, but be able to bend with the wind. A fit Wood element will manifest as a powerful leader and inspire those around them.

A person with an imbalanced Wood element will always be angry and frustrated, sensing that they are always stuck and never moving forward in life. Every experience is a fight. They are unable to grow.

They are total perfectionists who never get anything accomplished, because it has to be perfect.

What follows is a brief list of the functions of the liver and gallbladder in both Western and Chinese terms. As with all the organs discussed in this book, you'll see that sometimes there is an overlap. As a little reminder, Chinese medicine knew these functions centuries and even thousands of years before Western medicine "discovered" them. I've included Western functions both to give you a better understanding of how your body works (particularly when it's showing signs of distress), and also to help you figure out what imbalances you have to help heal any related emotion(s).

There are only a few similarities between Western functions of the liver and gallbladder and the Chinese perspective on these organs. In Chinese medicine the liver is one of the most important organs, because it's in charge of so many functions.

Functions of the Liver	
Western Medicine	**TCM**
Builds blood, cleans the blood, and detoxifies the body of harmful chemicals	Builds blood, cleans the blood, and detoxifies the body of harmful chemicals
Breaks down fats, converts sugar to energy, produces urea (the main substance of urine), some vitamins and minerals, and maintains a proper level of glucose (sugar) in the blood	Moves qi throughout the body, stores blood, regulates the menses by controlling how much blood goes into the uterus, and is connected to reproductive organs
Can be made toxic by fatty foods and alcohol	Can be made toxic by fatty foods, alcohol, and suppressed anger

What do I mean above by "harmful chemicals"? Unfortunately, even if you eat really clean, organic food and wear only organic clothes, you're being exposed to substances that make your liver work overtime. Alcohol, air and water pollution, fluoride, heavy metals and radiation, pesticides, medications, plastic, and chemicals in our clothes, paint, furniture, beauty products, and cleaning products all need to be filtered out by the liver. Pretty grim, I know. This constant exposure to toxins is why I recommend doing a liver cleanse at least once a year. If the liver is trying to process too many toxic substances, it can't flush all of them out. This can lead to a buildup of these toxins in the body, which causes added stress for the liver and can eventually lead to liver failure, liver cancer, and toxicity throughout the body.

In Eastern medicine, the liver channel is seen as wrapping around your reproductive organs. A possible manifestation of an imbalance in the liver is excess dampness and heat in the liver. This excess can cause herpes, infertility, ovarian cysts, or an enlarged prostate. These alone should be motivation enough to take care of your liver.

What do I mean by excess "dampness and heat"? The body has a naturally occurring amount of damp and heat in the body. Dampness keeps things moist and lubricated. Heat keeps us warm and aids in digestion. As with the balance of yin and yang you learned about in chapter 3, there's a fine line between the right amount and too much or too little. Too much dampness can lead to phlegm in the lungs; not enough can make your poop dry. Too much heat can cause burning urination; not enough can make your metabolism slow down. Our bodies are highly effective, extremely sensitive machines that need to be taken care of. I'm always amazed by how well they hold up even when we abuse them. It's time to start taking care of your body now.

If you know someone who is extremely judgmental, they probably have a gallbladder imbalance. What follows are the functions of the gallbladder, as seen from Eastern and Western perspectives.

Functions of the Gallbladder	
Western Medicine	**TCM**
Stores and excretes bile to break down fat	Stores and excretes bile to break down fat
	Making decisions, providing qi to the sinews for movement, and judgment

What does "providing qi to the sinews for movement" mean? If the gallbladder is imbalanced, you may experience awkward movements of your limbs or feel weak or strained when trying to move about. Imagine walking around and feeling like your legs have no energy. This could be from your gallbladder not being happy.

PHYSICAL SYMPTOMS

Each organ has several physical symptoms associated with its imbalance. I must reiterate that if your organ shows signs of distress in Chinese terms, *it doesn't mean the actual organ is affected.* So when I say the liver is imbalanced, weak, or deficient, I don't want you to think something is wrong with your physical liver. You don't need to think, *Oh my God! I need to get to the doctor now!* Relating to the functions of a particular organ is simply another tool for diagnosing and coming up with the best possible treatment.

The liver has the most related symptoms attached to it. Below is list of many of them.

- More than half my patients suffered from headaches on a regular basis before coming in for treatments. Headaches— either stabbing or aching at temples, vertex/crown, and/or behind eyes, migraines, high blood pressure, flank pain, and a red face—are your body's way of saying it's under some type of stress, and they are an indication of some type of imbalance. Causes may include stress, dehydration, food allergies, hormonal imbalances, high blood pressure, heavy metal poisoning, caffeine withdrawal, medication side effects, or a head cold.

- Because the liver controls blood going into the uterus, women with a liver imbalance may have gynecological problems, including heavy periods or a lot of cramping. PMS symptoms such as mood swings, water retention, and breast tenderness may be exacerbated, and women may also experience irregular menses and blood clots accompanying the period.

- Since the liver channel wraps around the genitals, men with liver issues may experience prostatitis, premature ejaculation, impotence, and/or infertility.

- Pain or temperature change along the liver channel may manifest as cancer, gallstones, cirrhosis, anemia, thrombosis/blood clotting, red eyes, blurry vision, floaters/seeing stars, dry eyes, brittle nails, or nail ridges/lines.

- Nervous system–related problems include vertigo, dizziness, Alzheimer's disease, Parkinson's disease, epilepsy, and strokes.

- Other general symptoms are possible: craving sour-tasting foods, dry/brittle hair, hair loss, premature gray, knots in the stomach, weak or tight joints/tendons/ligaments/muscles, low-pitched ringing in the ears, and muscle spasms.

As you can see, your liver plays a very important role in your overall health. Are you ready to pay better attention to it? I see a lot of my patients' symptoms disappear when we primarily focus on their liver. It seems that once you let go of the anger and resentment, a lot of discomfort is let go as well.

Compared with the liver, the gallbladder only has a few symptoms associated with it, which is typical for all yang organs. These include difficulty making decisions, pain and temperature change along the gallbladder channel, headaches at the temples, gallstones, shyness, belching, and nausea.

Dehydration

Most people I see in my clinic are dehydrated. You are supposed to drink approximately half your weight in ounces of water. This means if you weigh 140 pounds, you should be drinking approximately 70 ounces of water per day. This doesn't include the additional water necessary when you've been sweating, eaten, taken medications, or consumed beverages (coffee, tea, soda, alcohol) that make you lose even more water. Many headaches, muscle pain, and other health complaints would go away or be minimized if people just drank enough water. And here's an interesting fact: Dehydration can make you crave sugar. So for all you sugar junkies reading this, drink up! If you need help remembering to drink enough water, set an alarm on your phone to go off every two hours during your waking hours, and drink at least one glass every time the alarm sounds.

WHAT'S REALLY BEHIND YOUR CRAVINGS?

Cravings. We all have them. The question is why? Why for some things and not for others? And why is it they're usually for things that aren't healthy?

Dr. Doug Lisle and Alan Goldhamer's *The Pleasure Trap: Mastering the Hidden Force that Undermines Health & Happiness* goes into great detail about what actually happens to our brains when we want the bad stuff (or typically the bad stuff). In a nutshell, every time we feel good due to an experience or something we've consumed, new connections form in the brain asking for more. Just think of the thousands of chocolate-wanting neurons begging for more!

Also, our minds are designed to put in the least amount of effort for the biggest pleasure response. This definitely worked to our advantage before the agricultural age, when we foraged (and hunted) for food. We ate what we needed to survive. But now that we have easy access to way more food, and a big chunk of it is incredibly unhealthy, this primal instinct is slowly (or quickly) killing us. This chemical makeup in our brains can make us dependent on a whole host of things: sugar, salt, caffeine, dairy, or booze.

On top of that, processed and junk "food" is designed to make us addicted. Food scientists have this in mind with every ingredient they create and add to that can of soup, bag of flavored chips, McDonald's fries, or the flavored drinks most Americans consume daily. This makes it physically difficult to give up certain foods. Our bodies feel like they can't live without them. Even the *New York Times* featured an article about this very real Orwellian problem. Pretty disturbing.

One thing you won't see in this book is any suggestions for dessert. This isn't because I don't want you to have a treat. If you're going to eat something sweet, I prefer it in fruit form. And if you're eating out much or buying premade foods, soups, salad dressings, or sauces, you're eating too much sugar. The United States Department of Agriculture (USDA) recommends that people who eat 2,000 calories per day should limit their daily sugar intake to 10 teaspoons, or 42 grams. But most Americans eat about 21 teaspoons, or 88 grams per day. The American Heart Association recommends 6 to 9 teaspoons (25 to 38 grams), which I think is more like it. When it comes to sugar, less is always best.

You can also crave certain foods because you're lacking a nutrient found in that food. It might not be the best food for you, or even the best source, but your brain asks for it. If you've ever had to have a hamburger or steak, you might be lacking iron. That's really what you're craving. But there's no need to actually eat beef; you can pick up a kale salad, lentils, chickpeas, edamame, or tempeh. Make sure to eat C-rich foods or take vitamin C to aid in the absorption of iron. When you're dying for chocolate at that time of the month, you might be low in magnesium. Yes, it could be the sugar. But specifically craving chocolate when you're PMSing might be a deficiency issue; try pumpkin seeds, quinoa, almonds, oatmeal, spinach, black-eyed peas, or a baked potato instead. I often recommend a quality calcium and magnesium supplement to moderate cravings, which will also help reduce other PMS symptoms, including cramps. If you crave seafood, you may need more healthy fat in your diet. Make sure to eat some omega-3-rich sources daily—hemp, kale, flaxseeds, seaweed, or walnuts. Avocado is another fat fave of mine. That all encompassing "need" for dairy comes from casomorphin, an opiate-like chemical produced when digesting dairy products. It hooks you before you even realize it. For humans, cows, or goats, its real purpose is to make sure babies drink enough of their mother's milk.

We can also have an emotional attachment to certain foods and the memories that come with what Mom used to cook for us when we weren't feeling well. You may associate ice cream with having a reward. Or you may have a connection with certain holiday meals that can be hard to break. If you think that Thanksgiving just won't be the same without turkey, butter, sugar, or tons of wine, it may be hard to make a change. But there are plenty of healthier options and recipes available. Eventually, you won't miss it.

I recommend adding foods that will help you thrive. Get creative. Try something new every week or two. Your palate will change, and you'll start to crave more of the good stuff. It's also important not to see the changes as deprivation. Feeling like you're missing out on the joys of life will set you up to fail. Think of all the new foods you get to try and how much better you're feeling instead. If you're having a tough time saying no, then get help from friends and family, or even a support group. Having people around you who have been there is a great tool.

Should you give in to these cravings? Only you can truly answer that. For most people, indulging occasionally is a slippery slope.

WHAT? NO COFFEE?

Almost all of my patients regularly drink coffee when they first come to see me. And you know what they hate to give up as much as sugar? That's right, coffee. If you're a coffee drinker, you're not going to like what you're about to read. But this information is vital. Many think it's good for them. At least decaf isn't bad for you, right? Sorry! You want to know why I encourage them to give it up? Keep reading!

Toxicity

Caffeine combines with the stomach's hydrochloric acid to form a potent toxin: caffeine hydrochloride. When it's absorbed, bile is released in an attempt to flush the toxin from your system. This accounts for increased bowel regularity, of which many coffee drinkers boast. If you only have a bowel movement after your morning coffee, most likely your body has become dependent on the laxative side effect.

Decaffeinated coffee is no better, because it contains a large concentration of the chemical trichloroethylene. It is used mostly as a degreasing agent in the metal industry and as a dry cleaning agent. It is linked to liver cancer.

Adrenal Exhaustion

Coffee stimulates your adrenal glands to secrete adrenaline, which activates your fight-or-flight response. This stimulates insulin secretion and leads to secondary hypoglycemia, which results in a mild rise in blood pressure, a craving for sweets two to three hours later, low energy and mood, and overworking the adrenals.

Nutritional Deficiencies

Drinking coffee and tea reduces iron absorption by 40 to 60 percent, thereby increasing the risk of anemia.

Osteoporosis

Coffee also raises the acidity levels of your blood, causing calcium to be pulled from your bones and teeth to use as a buffering agent. This puts you at an even greater risk for osteoporosis and kidney stones.

Other Side Effects

Some other adverse effects of drinking coffee include insomnia, tremors, anxiety, restlessness, irritability, headaches, temporary increase in the stiffening of arterial walls, elevated blood pressure and/or cholesterol levels, irregular heartbeat and palpitations, increased risk of a heart attack, PMS symptoms, increased risk of bladder and rectal cancer, and higher risk of the birth of a low-birth-weight child.

Caffeine is a very strong diuretic (it makes you pee). Most coffee drinkers are dehydrated, which can result in electrolyte imbalances, kidney failure, and confusion (even coma) due to decreased blood flow to organs and the brain.

I know the thought of giving up your morning coffee sounds almost impossible, and that could be because caffeine belongs to the same alkaloid group as morphine, cocaine, and strychnine. But think of how much better you'll feel once you've quit. The initial withdrawal symptoms and crankiness will subside. If you're worried about being tired at work, then slowly make the switch to green tea or kombucha (a healthier drink for energy and health). It will be worth it.

CASE STUDIES

Below are two examples of patients I treated who had a predominance of liver issues, both physical and mental. This should help you better understand what it means to have liver disharmony. Having the whole story instead of just a list of symptoms should make it even easier to understand the concepts of TCM and how mental health reflects in physical health.

Jennifer

When Jennifer first walked in, I could see she was in a lot of physical pain. She carried herself in a way that said she was hesitant to move. Jennifer was thirty-nine years old, single, about fifty pounds overweight, and unable to work due to work-related injuries that lead to carpal tunnel syndrome. She'd seen a chiropractor a couple of times for the pain with minimal results. Jennifer had heard about my success treating carpal tunnel syndrome and weight issues through a friend, and decided to give me a try.

Her pain was the main, if not only, reason she initially came to see me. But once I read her intake form and asked her a few questions, I could tell there were several other issues we had to address. As I mentioned earlier, Chinese medicine treats not only the symptoms but also the root cause of an illness or injury to truly heal the problem. So Jennifer was the perfect candidate for TCM.

When I asked how she was doing emotionally with the amount of discomfort she was experiencing, Jennifer was pretty open. She admitted to having a very short fuse, and she also tended to worry quite a bit about her condition. These behaviors weren't new for her, but they'd definitely amplified in the last few months. Jennifer also had a history of mild depression and a pattern of not speaking up for herself.

She was also very judgmental, which can be a sign of a liver imbalance. Even on her first visit, she spent half the time complaining about how everyone around her was doing something wrong. Even the mailman didn't deliver her mail the right way, in her opinion.

Jennifer was one of those patients who wanted to get better but was holding back and feeling stuck. She'd tried every diet and always gained the weight back; she said she was tired of the yo-yo dieting and the lack of lasting results. Jennifer was a perfectionist and felt that if she wasn't eating precisely the right foods all the time she shouldn't bother. Years of therapy seemed to only be a temporary fix for her lifelong low-grade depression. Any sort of setback at work or in her personal life would bring the melancholy and overeating right back.

Pain made her sleep erratic. Sometimes painkillers knocked her out, and she'd fall asleep as soon as her head hit the pillow. Other times, Jennifer tried to take a break from her medication because it made her feel so out of it, but this made it hard to fall asleep. She slept well for the most part, except for the three to five nights before her period; then she had difficulty falling asleep and experienced nightmares. Jennifer mentioned that she often had dreams about fighting and yelling at strangers. The nights she had these dreams, she would wake up feeling full of resentment toward her family.

Jennifer had several other liver symptoms, including migraines, muscle tension in her back and neck, adult acne, premature graying, red eyes, and high blood pressure. I knew without a doubt that treating her liver, along with employing specific acupoints in an acupuncture treatment, would give her the best possible results.

We know that extra weight is an issue for general health. However, another way to look at it is that excess weight leads to inflammation all over the body, which increases pain. So we had to address her eating habits to help her physical health as well. Jennifer said she tried to eat healthy, but tended to overeat and consumed too many sweets. Her sugar cravings increased when experiencing PMS. She said she felt like she was possessed when PMSing, that something took over her brain and made her eat ridiculous amounts of lemon tarts and sorbet. She would hoard Sour Patch Kids like they were being discontinued. I'm sure many women reading this can relate.

My treatments and dietary suggestions focused on her initial complaint—pain resulting from carpal tunnel syndrome. There are plenty of foods that have anti-inflammatory qualities, including peas, asparagus, cucumber, and pumpkin. Actually, most fruits and veggies will reduce inflammation.

One of the great things about Chinese medicine is that you can address several concerns in one treatment. The same goes with herbal remedies. So not only did I treat her pain, but I worked on the other issues as well. Since many of her symptoms were connected to her liver, I used acupuncture points to support the liver.

I also gave dietary suggestions to help heal the liver. With all case studies in this book, I provide a sample meal plan of what I suggested. Keep in mind that Jennifer's plan is catered to her needs. You'll be able to make your own lists with the help of the other information you learn in this book.

Here is one of my sample meal plans for Jennifer. As you can see, nothing is too complicated or hard to make. Of course more seasoned chefs who have plenty of time to spend in the kitchen can make their meals more elaborate. But as I've written before, I try to be realistic in my suggestions. Who has two hours to spend on cooking dinner every night? Note that for all my patients I also recommend adding lemon to their water, especially first thing in the morning. It gets the intestines working, alkalizes the body, and aids in absorption of water.

Breakfast: smoothie with cherries, peaches, strawberries, unsweetened rice milk, chia seeds, and Vega One powder. (Vega One powder is one of the best protein powders on the market. It's not only high in protein from pea, hemp seeds, and brown rice, but it's packed full of vital nutrients from whole foods including broccoli, spinach, chlorella, pomegranate, and chia and flax seeds.)

Lunch: salad with sprouts, lettuce, celery, cucumber, kale, hemp seeds, and turnips, in a lemon juice–based dressing with garlic and spices; lentil soup with leeks.

Snacks: grapes, blackberries, sunflower seeds, plums, or an unsweetened trail mix with cherries and nuts.

Dinner: brown rice with steamed kale and broccoli, raw fermented cabbage, shredded ginger.

Jennifer's improvements were impressive. Her carpal tunnel improved about 25 percent in a couple of months, but Jennifer ended up opting for surgery. Her primary care physician and pain management specialist encouraged this, and I understood—she just wanted to be done with the pain. As with most conditions, I can't be certain what kind of results my patients will experience. All of them do get at least some relief. But sometimes the relief isn't happening fast enough. I encourage my patients to give their healing process some time. We're so used to the quick fix of Western medicine, however, it can be difficult to wait for the lasting results of healing the root cause.

Not only did her carpal tunnel symptoms improve, but Jennifer also felt better in general. Her hair became much thicker, and the gray started to disappear. Her blood pressure lowered dramatically and was consistently in normal range within weeks of starting acupuncture. She also mentioned that she felt less stressed and depressed since coming for acupuncture. As she started to get better, she also no longer felt the need to judge other people or herself so harshly. Jennifer realized she doesn't have to do everything exactly right, which took a lot pressure off of her.

Jennifer noticed remarkable improvement with her PMS symptoms. She was less irritable and was eating a lot less raspberry sorbet and chocolate. Outside of PMS mode, her mood improved quite a bit. Jennifer said her treatments with me helped her let go of a lot of her rage, and she had started forgiving the people she felt had hurt her. The low-level depression started to lift. She described herself as feeling lighter. Even friends and family commented on how laid-back she had become.

Jennifer admitted to following my nutritional guidelines about 50 percent of the time. She would make changes for two or three days, then slowly go back to eating the foods she was used to. Every time she saw me, she was reinspired to eat better. I appreciated her honesty on this. I let my patients know that I'm not judging them if they slip back into old habits. I've been there. I had such an addiction to dairy that it took me over twenty years of trying to give it up before I actually did. Being honest about where you're at and what you're doing can only help your practitioner help you.

I've been told by several of my patients that when they're tempted to eat or buy something they know they shouldn't, they picture me or someone else who motivates them encouraging them to make smart choices. I didn't come up with this idea myself. Several of my patients have said they did this, and it helped them to stay on track. Of course, this visualization doesn't always work, but it's nice to know I have had that much of an impact.

I'm confident that Jennifer would have had even better success with her treatments if she had stuck with it a bit longer. Since her treatments were covered by worker's compensation insurance, she was unable to see me after she opted to have the surgery. I heard from her about a year after her surgery, and she said that her pain reduced another 30 percent after the procedure.

Recap of Jennifer's Wood-related symptoms: muscle pain, migraines, irritability, depression, premature gray hair, high blood pressure, high cholesterol, anger in dreams, PMS, being judgmental.

Kevin

Suppressing anger can manifest as liver imbalances in so many ways. Kevin's story is another great example of how holding on to frustration and resentment can impact your physical health.

I knew Kevin was stressed from the moment I met him. He wasn't the worse case I've ever treated—unfortunately, far from it. But he gave off that vibe of "I'm about to lose it." Kevin was a fifty-eight-year-old male, married with three grown children, an accountant, and was referred to me by a patient who had also suffered from high blood pressure.

All my patients fill out a detailed medical intake form when first coming to see me. Kevin listed several chief complaints on his initial visit with me, which is another sign of someone being stressed. Usually, "chief complaint" means one major health concern; occasionally, people include a second ailment in this category. Kevin's chief complaints on his intake form were high blood pressure, glaucoma, high cholesterol, and benign tremors. He didn't know this at the time, but all of these are liver symptoms. For some of them he was taking Western medication and was told by his doctors that these meds would be necessary his entire life. Most of them were helping only slightly, some none at all, and Kevin was very concerned about the side effects.

On top of all that, Kevin had quite a list of other physical complaints: environmental allergies, constipation, headaches behind the eyes, bloating, indigestion, red eyes with yellow sclera (whites of the eyes), and weight gain only in his belly. Gaining weight only in the belly is often caused by stress. The adrenal glands release a hormone called cortisol whenever you are stressed, exhausted, or overwhelmed, and elevated cortisol levels tell the body to make more belly fat.

While getting to know Kevin over the course of several weeks, I noticed that he was very frustrated with several aspects of his life: his marriage, family dynamics, work, money, and living situation. Kevin felt that people around him prevented him from being happy. He held resentment toward several family members, and he also got pretty angry when discussing his past. When I saw Kevin, he was often annoyed and irritated about some aspect of his life.

Low energy levels were a major concern for Kevin. He was so tired at the end of the day that he would pass out as soon as his head hit the pillow. He also didn't remember any of his dreams. Even after a solid eight hours, Kevin felt exhausted and drank three cups of coffee just to be able to get up and get out of the house. In Kevin's case, his fatigue came from a host of reasons: caffeine dependency, poor diet, side effects of medications, and stress.

And talk about poor eating habits and needing to make some changes. Kevin ate the Standard American Diet (SAD), consisting of fast food, coffee, soda, meat, dairy, white bread, minimal veggies, nothing organic, and almost no water. I'm still amazed that the body can survive, albeit not very well, for decades eating like this.

With everyone I see, I make sure my dietary suggestions are realistic. Unless someone tells me they're totally ready for a complete overhaul or they're very sick (cancer, morbidly obese, AIDS), I keep it simple. This gradual shift in eating habits makes it more likely you'll keep doing it and you won't feel deprived in any way. One of the reasons extreme and fad diets don't work is that they aren't sustainable. Some personalities work well with going cold turkey on everything at once, but I rarely see this.

I gave Kevin several options for liver-boosting foods, encouraging him to gradually add some of them into his diet. Like most people, he originally wasn't very happy to hear the suggestions. But right away he did drink less soda, had a few glasses of water per day, and tried what he considered "healthy fast food," which isn't healthy at all. But he was at least motivated to make changes and was open to suggestions. Over the years, as he felt better, he became more and more motivated to improve his eating habits. After a few years Kevin gave up all fast food, stopped soda and coffee, and only ate seafood a couple of times a year. See, slow and steady does win the race.

The Joys of Hummus

I recommend hummus or some version of it to most people. Why? Because it's a healthy, easy-to-make (or buy) snack or sandwich spread. You can't really go wrong with hummus, unless you're allergic to one of its ingredients; if so, you just modify the recipe to suit your needs. It's high in fiber, protein, calcium, manganese, copper, and also has some calcium, iron, magnesium, and zinc. It is relatively rich in vitamins C and B_6, and also contains vitamin E, vitamin K, folate, and thiamin. It's also low in sugar and carbohydrates.

There were some long-term goals I had for Kevin. More water. Less coffee and eventually no coffee except for an occasional treat. No soda. No fast food. Fresh veggies daily. I suggested he incorporate them one at time, or let go of the habits one by one. Once he felt stable with one of them, he did one more. With most patients this process takes anywhere from a week to a month.

Kevin's meal plan consisted of healthier versions of foods he liked. Burritos with tons of meat, cheese, and sour cream became wraps with rice, veggies, and avocado.

Breakfast: juice with kale, beets, celery, apple, and ginger; oatmeal with flaxseeds and berries if he was still hungry.

Lunch: whole grain Ezekiel or brown rice bread with lots of veggies (sprouts, tomato, cucumber, lettuce, shredded carrots, and beets), mustard, Daiya cheese, and tempeh; or a rice tortilla with lots of roasted veggies, brown rice, and guacamole.

Snacks: rice crackers or celery and carrot sticks with nut butter, babaganoush, or hummus; chamomile tea for stress reduction throughout the day.

Dinner: quinoa pasta with tomato sauce, veggies, and tempeh "meatballs."

Talk about progress! Kevin's cholesterol dropped thirty points in one month. After eight months his cholesterol levels were at a very healthy 145. Along with that his blood pressure was a healthy 115 over 82, and his glaucoma was gone within three months. The hand tremors reduced about 30 percent. He and his doctor couldn't believe the results, especially because he had achieved them without cholesterol or blood-pressure medication. Kevin was always commenting on how much easier he was able to handle stress. He was fighting less with his wife. He thought that his mood and attitude would never improve before coming to see me. He was amazed by the calmness that became a part of his daily life. Kevin said that if I had told him what his life would be like in less than a year, he wouldn't have believed me.

Recap of Kevin's Wood-related symptoms: high blood pressure, short fuse, stress, yellow sclera, fatigue, tremors, high cholesterol.

There are plenty of delicious foods to help harmonize the liver. Probably most of you reading this section have at least a few of the liver symptoms. But now you see how many great options there are. You feel satisfied with all the variety and amazing tastes.

With all that you've learned about suppressing anger and resentment and its impact on your well-being, you now have some tools to heal. Do you think you have a compromised liver? The examples I shared should give you some ideas of what to eat to heal your liver and release any suppressed emotions. Whether it's PMS or high cholesterol, you can fix it with food.

When the heart is at ease, the body is healthy.

—Chinese Proverb

CHAPTER 8

Heartbreaker

Matters of the Heart

Recommended Foods

For heart complaints in general, these foods are good: corn, shiitake mushrooms, whole wheat, brown rice, green beans, peanuts, pears, oats, garbanzo beans, beets, mulberries, lemon, pomegranate, dill, basil, chamomile, marjoram, bell peppers, celery, lettuce, romaine lettuce, cucumbers (with skin), and tomatoes.

Not having enough qi in the heart is pretty common. Overexercising is one of the main causes of heart qi deficiency. **For palpitations on exertion, fatigue, muscle weakness, sweating without exertion, and lowered heart rate while exercising (all symptoms of heart qi deficiency),** eat these foods: cinnamon, carrots, daikon radishes, red radishes, saffron, onions, garlic, and cherries.

Not enough yang in an organ usually manifests as qi deficiency plus some sense of being cold. **For palpitations, cold limbs or feeling cold, fatigue, and spontaneous sweating (all symptoms of heart yang deficiency),** try the qi-fortifying foods listed above, plus walnuts, chives, cayenne pepper, raspberries, strawberries, blueberries, blackberries, ginger, clove, and cardamom.

Heart blood deficiency means there isn't enough healthy blood flowing through the heart. This isn't the same as having a heart attack, with a complete lack of blood flow or when the heart stops pumping. **For palpitations, insomnia, nightmares, anxiety, being easily startled, dizziness, pale lips/complexion, poor long-term memory, and inability to concentrate (all symptoms of heart blood deficiency),** eat as many of these as possible: yams, sweet potatoes, parsnips, turnips, pumpkin, millet, spelt, cherries, grapes, butternut squash, beets, onions, leeks, garlic, parsley, chard, kale, and bok choy.

When the heart doesn't have enough yin, it can lead to a whole host of issues. **For night sweats, hot flashes, palpitations, insomnia, nightmares, anxiety, startling easily, dry mouth, and poor long-term memory (all symptoms of heart yin deficiency),** try these foods often: fava, mung, and kidney beans, persimmons, apples, black sesame seeds, flaxseeds, seaweed, peaches, blueberries, blackberries, mangoes, bananas, coconut, endive, and asparagus.

The heart isn't meant to have any phlegm in it at all. **For palpitations, mental illnesses, thirst, red face, bitter taste in mouth in morning, dark urine, phlegm, insomnia, nightmares, restlessness, and manic behavior (all symptoms of heart phlegm),** these are beneficial foods: kale, collard greens, mustard greens, ginger, seaweed, and bamboo shoots.

All of the foods recommended above support the Fire element.

Foods to Avoid or Minimize

For heart yin deficiency: cinnamon, coffee, vinegar, shellfish, garlic, leeks, and peppers

For heart phlegm: nuts, seeds, dairy, and grains

Have you ever had your heart broken? Do you remember how you felt? Did you feel like you would never recover? Sometimes the aftermath can be so bad that friends and family think about doing an intervention, or you feel like having yourself committed. The effects of feeling like your heart has been ripped to shreds can include anxiety; the inability to eat, sleep, or think; chest pain; fatigue; depression; and weight loss or gain.

Have you felt all of the above and maybe much more? Heartache can come from romantic love, a loss of a friend or companion, or a shock such as being hurt or betrayed by someone you love.

It is said that you can die from a broken heart. You've probably heard the stories of an elderly couple who had been together for decades dying within months of each other. Well, in TCM this makes complete sense. When you've had a big shock or had your heart broken, it can deplete your heart's qi to the point where it actually stops beating. A great emotional shock to the heart, usually from the death of a long-term spouse, drastically depletes the heart of its qi. Without enough qi, the heart, or any organ, for that matter, can't function anymore.

In Western terms, the physical pain we've all experienced can come from a rush of adrenaline or other hormones, leading to decreased blood flow to the heart or stunning the heart into not pumping properly. This lack of blood leads to chest pain. That's why a breakup can physically hurt so damn much. It's not your imagination. Physiologically there's something happening.

The Fire element is associated with the heart and small intestines and opens to the tongue. This element is also associated with summer. Fire is about passion and being dynamic. When the Fire element is strong, you can easily experience joy, laughter, love, and an eagerness to live life. You can share love unconditionally and easily with a balanced Fire element. You can effortlessly share kindness and compassion with those around you, even if you don't really like them. If you have a healthy Fire element, even having your heart broken by someone you love won't hurt as much or last as long. You intuitively know with whom it is safe to be vulnerable.

When Fire is weak you might be emotionally sensitive or cold, or very insecure when it comes to love and love relationships. You can be passionless, easily hurt, or even codependent. A fragile Fire element can also result in the constant fear of rejection. Someone who manically talks, laughs inappropriately, and is always telling jokes has a compromised Fire element.

Opening to or affecting the tongue, as you learned earlier, means that if you're experiencing a heart imbalance, you may have issues with your speech. This includes muteness, lisps, a "cat got your tongue" feeling, and stuttering. If you have experienced true heartache, you can probably remember a few instances when you felt like you couldn't get your words out.

As the chart below shows, there is some overlap in functions when comparing Western and Chinese theory. But the heart has a whole host of functions in TCM that Westerners don't normally connect to it.

Functions of the Heart	
Western Medicine	**TCM**
Regulates and promotes circulation of oxygenated blood throughout the body	Regulates blood flow
Removes waste	Regulates sleep and houses your mind/soul
	Controls sweat
	Sends heat to bladder and uterus
	Stimulates small intestine function

The heart is considered the king of all the organs in TCM. It is necessary to keep the heart healthy and happy to guarantee the health of the rest of the body. Without maintaining its optimal function, a person cannot live a full life mentally, emotionally, spiritually, or physically. The heart regulates blood flow throughout the body, into every cell, regulates the amount and quality of sleep, houses your soul/mind, provides warmth to the spleen, stimulates the function of separation in the small intestines, and sends heat to the bladder so that it can excrete fluids (make you pee). Pay attention to your urination if you experience insomnia. Burning urination upon waking might be the result of your heart sending too much heat to the bladder or small intestine during the night. And if the heart is imbalanced, it will show up in some way on the face, perhaps a blemish, change in color, or a skin condition.

What do I mean when I say that the heart "houses the soul"? It is a Chinese belief that our soul or consciousness rests in the heart at night while we're sleeping. That is the main reason that any issues with the heart will likely show up as insomnia and/or mental health complaints. The mind needs a safe, cozy place to go for some down-time. It needs plenty of rest to function well. Think about the last time you couldn't sleep. How cranky were you the next day? Imagine having chronic insomnia and what that would do to your mental state.

The heart also provides warmth to the spleen to aid in digestion. It stimulates the function of separation in the small intestines. Too much heat in the heart can lead to abdominal pain, sudden loss of hearing, and burning urination. The heart also sends heat to the uterus to keep blood moving. Not enough heat can manifest as menstrual cramps or the lack of a period, or with too much heat quite the opposite: heavy bleeding.

The heart controls sweat, which is very obvious when someone having a heart attack begins to sweat profusely—usually an oily type of sweat. Unexplained spontaneous sweating can be caused if there is not enough qi in the heart.

The small intestine is the yang-paired organ to the heart. It relies on the heart's heat to aid in metabolism. "Small intestine" is a funny name for something that averages about twenty feet long. It is actually much longer than the large intestine, which is typically about five feet long but gets its name because of its width: The small intestine is typically one-third the width of the large intestine.

As with all yang organs, there are just a few symptoms related to an imbalanced small intestine. Among them are difficulty determining right from wrong, burning urination upon waking, abdominal pain, sudden hearing loss, gas, vomiting, and either scanty or excessive urine. The small intestines can also have parasites.

The emotions associated with the small intestines are similar to the heart, with the additional ability to determine right from wrong. So small children, whose small intestines are still developing, need guidance as to what is "bad" and "good." Dishonest people can still have healthy small intestines even if they know what they're doing is wrong. Some of these people are called psychopaths; they do bad things but have no conscience, or they even get pleasure from harming others.

In Western medicine the small intestine absorbs nutrients and removes waste. In TCM it serves to separate the impure from the pure. It can help eliminate physical impurity—waste or toxins—but also emotional impurity. This makes it unique. For example, when someone says something negative to you, such as "I hate you," the small intestine takes that negative message and keeps it away from the heart. The heart will then be protected from any damage. In TCM, harmful words and actions, not just harmful foods and substances, can hurt an organ. The heart is the most vulnerable, which is why the small intestines, along with the pericardium, protect it.

Susan, one of my patients featured a little later in this chapter, is the poster child for this issue. She is what is called an empath. Empaths are highly sensitive and feel everything, sometimes to an extreme. They are naturally very giving and good listeners. When empaths absorb the impact of stressful emotions, it can trigger panic attacks; depression; food, sex, and drug binges; and a plethora of physical symptoms. Susan definitely takes on other people's pain and baggage. This is probably a contributing factor to her drug addiction.

There are several emotions associated with the heart in TCM, even more than the liver, which sort of makes sense to our Western minds, doesn't it? The heart is where physically we feel our feelings, where we love, ache, grieve, and feel joy.

Lack of joy, excitability, anxiety, heartbreak, long-term memory loss, depression, and mental illness are all symptoms of an imbalanced heart. All of these examples can be temporary or more chronic, mild or severe in nature.

The physical signs of an imbalanced heart are mostly connected to the actual (physical) heart, and there are fewer symptoms than for any other yin organ. They include angina/chest pain, heart disease, heart attacks, epilepsy, encephalitis, irregular heartbeat, stuttering, palpitations, bitter taste in the morning, pain or temperature change along the heart channel, aphasia (inability to speak), muteness, shortness of breath when exercising, poor long-term memory, menopausal symptoms (the kidneys can also cause menopause symptoms), and arrhythmia.

Palpitations involve an irregularity of the heartbeat. They can manifest either as a rapid or slow pulse or skipped beats, which can lead to difficulty breathing. They are generally not dangerous if there is no underlying heart disease. Non-heart-related causes of palpitations include illegal drugs, certain legal drugs that stress the heart, alcohol, caffeine, nicotine, vigorous physical activity, stress, panic attacks, anxiety, low electrolyte or blood-sugar levels, dehydration, thyroid disorders, low blood pressure, anemia, and some herbal/nutritional supplements. Female hormonal changes can also lead to palpitations, particularly those that occur during pregnancy, menopause, perimenopause, or menstruation.

If you've ever experienced palpitations, you know they can be pretty scary and uncomfortable. Can you imagine having them every day for months?

A big chunk of symptoms related to the heart involve mental illness. These include bipolar disorder/manic depression, schizophrenia, addiction, borderline personality disorder, panic attacks, rash/impulsive behavior, laughing for no reason, attention deficit disorder (ADD) and/or attention deficit/hyperactivity disorder (ADHD), obsessive(OCD), autism, insomnia, and nightmares.

CASE STUDIES

Since a majority of my patients come to me for mood enhancement and/or addiction, I have a plethora of case studies from which to choose for this section. Rick and Susan both had addictions and mental health problems, which is really no coincidence, because most addicts are self-medicating some type of mood disorder. This means people who have issues with depression, anxiety, or even more severe issues like schizophrenia often will reach for a drug, drink, and/or food to suppress and temporarily alleviate their emotional pain. This never fixes the problem and can lead to addiction.

Rick

When he first came in for treatment, Rick's main health concern was heart palpitations. He'd been experiencing them for eight months, and they had been occurring daily for three months. He had every imaginable test done on his heart and thyroid, and everything came back fine. Rick also had no history of panic attacks or recent drug use (apart from caffeine), so those were also ruled out. Previously Rick had been smoking marijuana daily to reduce his stress levels at night, but he stopped once the palpitations got severe. He wanted to see if his drug use was contributing to or causing his problem, but his symptoms did not change when he quit. (Note that for some people, marijuana can cause palpitations.) Rick wasn't taking any medications. He was a forty-two-year-old married lawyer with no children who worked sixty hours per week.

Rick had a few other medical issues, all of which he felt he could live with. But I wanted to know about them to get a complete picture of what was going on. Having all the information enables me to give the best diagnoses and treatment plans. He had constipation, gas and bloating, dry skin, low back pain, and painful, burning urination upon waking. Tests showed no infection or prostate problems that might be causing the urination issues.

Rick had nightmares regularly and experienced difficulty falling asleep nightly most of his life. His single mother was bipolar, and the result was a very unstable upbringing. Rick said he'd tried melatonin and other natural supplements without much success. He tried sleeping pills for a couple of weeks; they knocked him out, but he woke up after four hours and felt out of it the next day. This affected his work, so he stopped taking them.

From the first time we spoke, I knew Rick had some emotional issues. Even over the phone, he was very pushy about my accommodating his schedule. Rick expected me to come in after hours and on my days off for him. When I couldn't, he felt like it was a personal affront. His demeanor with me was aggressive and he got very angry when I reminded him he needed to be on time for his appointments (he was late for every appointment). Unfortunately, I had to let him go after twelve weeks due to his erratic behavior. I learned that at age forty he had been diagnosed with borderline personality disorder, which accounted for much of his behavior.

According to the National Institutes of Health, "borderline personality disorder (BPD) is a serious mental illness characterized by pervasive instability in moods, interpersonal relationships, self-image, and behavior. A person with BPD may experience intense bouts of anger, depression, and anxiety that may last only hours, or at most a day. These may be associated with episodes of impulsive aggression, self-injury, and drug or alcohol abuse." (I am specifically citing this disorder here because few people know about it. Psychiatric professionals have tried to treat BPD with some combination of medications and therapy, with mixed results.)

Rick's issues with scheduling may have been related to his BPD. He also mentioned the dynamics of his marriage and how unfair his wife was to him. When asked for an example of his wife's unfairness, his answers seemed insignificant: She was unable to remember that he hated blueberries and loved Britney Spears. Small slights such as these made him feel like she didn't really love him.

As with a majority of my patients, Rick ate a SAD diet. His standard routine included fast food, minimal water, five cups of coffee daily, no fresh fruits or vegetables, microwaved meals, cookies, and cakes. And following a pattern that has become all too common, none of his Western doctors had asked a single question about his eating habits.

Luckily, Rick was willing to try new things to get better. The palpitations scared him so much that he was starting to get desperate. He took Chinese herbs three times a day, had biweekly acupuncture, and revamped his diet. My nutritional advice started with the usual recommendations for SAD eaters: Drink more water, give up fast food and sugar, and reduce caffeine intake. For the time Rick was under my care, he was able to reduce his caffeine intake to only one cup of coffee per day. He had headaches at first and was a bit tired, but that improved after a few weeks. Within three weeks he was drinking six cups of water per day, a huge improvement for someone who previously drank at most one glass a day. Rick also cut out all refined sugar in six weeks, although he had a hard time giving up fast food and was still eating it several times per week—but he did add fruits to his breakfast and a salad every few days.

His meal plan was pretty simple. Here's an example of what I suggested for him:

Breakfast: oatmeal with banana, tahini, and hemp milk.

Lunch: enchiladas with kidney beans, scallions, red bell pepper, garlic, brown rice, and corn tortillas.

Snacks: celery sticks and hummus.

Dinner: salad with cucumber, celery, lettuce, mushrooms, radish, and bell pepper, and a creamy tomato soup with dill. (My favorite tomato soup recipe is super easy to make! Use onion, garlic, tomato, miso broth, and cashews. You can add either basil or dill, depending on which you prefer. Puree the cashews with either water or unsweetened nut milk before adding to simmering soup. Simmer for 15 minutes, and it's done.)

Rick saw many of his symptoms alleviated, even within a few months. I suspected caffeine, dehydration, and stress as the three main causes of his heart palpitations, and cutting back on caffeine and drinking more water helped tremendously. Rick's low back pain was minimized as well. This was primarily due to the increase in water (he was very dehydrated) and stronger adrenals after reducing his coffee intake. He also became less aggressive (typical in borderline personality disorder patients as a result of acupuncture), but he was still too much for me to handle. I hope Rick stuck with his new, healthy lifestyle.

Recap of Rick's Fire symptoms: palpitations, borderline personality disorder, burning urination, insomnia.

Susan

I've seen all kinds of mental illness cases and have heard some horrible stories over the years—starting during my internship in a psychiatric unit at a local hospital—so not much can faze me. Yes, I still feel compassion for all my patients and what they're going through, but it's rare that someone's story completely shocks me anymore (I don't know if this is a good thing or a bad thing). But Susan's story definitely knocked me for a loop.

Susan was referred to me by one of her friends who had been my patient and had gotten relief from lifelong depression. He was hopeful I could help Susan as well. I didn't know anything about her background, until he brought her to my office. Susan was a fifty-three-year-old recent widow with no children. Her chief complaint was daily panic attacks, which had been going on for six months. She had been hospitalized four times because her anti-anxiety medication wasn't helping. On several occasions Susan felt like she was having a heart attack, which can be a symptom of panic attacks.

Quantity and Quality

In the hectic, fast-paced world we live in, most of us don't get enough sleep. It may be because there aren't enough hours in the day, or kids keep you awake, or you're thinking about all the things that need to get done. Sleep is key to a healthy body and mind, and sleep quality is just as important as the amount of sleep. Taking sleeping pills doesn't help the quality at all. Without enough good sleep, you can be more prone to illness, injury, and elevated stress levels. Keep in mind that alcohol, caffeine, sleeping pills, and some medications can lead to unrestful sleep. If you're tired after a solid eight hours, something else may be going on with your health.

Lack of quality sleep can lead to the following conditions:

- **Weight gain:** Chronic insomnia can cause weight gain by elevating cortisol (stress hormone) levels, which stimulate fat production. How we process and store carbohydrates can be compromised as well.

- **Cardiovascular problems:** Insomnia may cause hypertension and irregular heartbeat.

- **Poor memory:** Sleep helps the brain commit new information to memory.

- **Mood issues:** Lack of sleep can cause anxiety, irritability, and poor concentration.

- **Illness:** Poor sleep weakens our immunity, making us more prone to illness. Getting enough rest is also vital to fighting cancer.

So turn off the TV and computer early, take a relaxing bath, drink some herbal tea, and get into bed. And sweet dreams.

In addition to experiencing severe heartbreak related to the recent, violent death of her husband, Susan had witnessed his murder, during which she had also been threatened. Can you imagine going through that? No wonder she was having a hard time coping! Although she was no longer in any danger, she still felt like it. Her body was in constant fight-or-flight mode.

The first time I saw Susan, she cried the entire session. Because she was so distraught, I only asked her a few key questions about her general health and gave her a treatment specifically for trauma. She was calmer within minutes, and I was able to find out about some of her other medical issues. Susan also had menopause symptoms and burning urination upon waking up. She was addicted to cocaine and had been for almost twenty years. Susan also had severe insomnia and sweated through her pajamas every night. Her inability to sleep more than three hours a night was partly emotional, partly due to menopause, and partly due to her use of cocaine. Somehow all of the medications Susan was taking didn't seem to help. Her medicine cabinet was a mini pharmacy. She had been on Xanax, Klonopin, Celexa, and Ambien for as long as she could remember, and she had upped the dosage on all of them since her husband's passing.

Susan didn't have much of an appetite due to the cocaine use and stress. She admitted to not eating more than one meal per day. Even before the death of her husband, she had almost no desire to eat, and when she did eat, it was mostly sweets, refined carbohydrates, and coffee. She rarely ate any whole foods or vegetables. Even though she ate very little, Susan had some issues with weight gain. I concluded it was mainly because her metabolism had slowed down due to thirty years without proper exercise, as well as insufficient nutrients and calories.

That first week Susan received four acupuncture sessions, then we gradually cut back as she felt calmer. I gave her a patented herbal formula to address her panic attacks and help her sleep, and encouraged her to seek help with her addiction, recent trauma and loss, and mental health issues.

Initially Susan was not ready to improve her diet. I didn't push her on this, because I was so concerned with her mental health. I did suggest trying to have a smoothie for breakfast to at least start off the day right, and suggested a meal plan for when she became more stable. It only took a few treatments and daily herbs before Susan made some big improvements.

My goal with Susan, and all my patients, is to give them realistic goals and lifestyle changes. Doing too much at once usually ends in failure and patients beating themselves up for that failure. That's one main reason why extreme diets rarely work. You feel you're being deprived of all the good things in life, and with some diets you end up limiting your caloric intake so much that it becomes unhealthy. As soon as you stop, you gain all the weight back and more. Then the guilt of not keeping it off or sticking to the diet makes it even worse.

I kept Susan's dietary suggestions very simple. Susan knew that eating better would help her mental state, so she was somewhat motivated to make some improvements.

Breakfast: smoothie with almond, hazelnut, or hemp milk, or coconut kefir with strawberries, raspberries, flaxseeds, tahini, or almond butter; a pomegranate or pomegranate juice.

Lunch: whole grain Ezekiel or brown rice bread, lots of veggies, no mustard, Daiya cheese, tempeh or eggless tofu salad, or a rice tortilla with lots of veggies, brown rice, and guacamole.

Snacks: unsweetened trail mix, black sesame rice crackers, or celery and carrot sticks with nut butter, babaganoush, tofu salad, or hummus.

Dinner: green salad with miso dressing or oil and lemon (no vinegar); any veggies plus sesame, pumpkin, sunflower, and/or hemp seeds; lots of sprouts; baked sweet potato or yam; steamed spinach with garlic and a little olive oil; quinoa or red rice with sautéed veggies.

Susan's progress, as with all my anxiety patients, was drastic. From the first treatment, when she immediately calmed down and stopped crying, her heart rate slowed and she was able to breathe. That first week she had only two mild anxiety attacks and no full-blown panic attacks. After six weeks she stopped taking all of her medications except Ambien and had only mild anxiety when she thought about her husband. No more panic attacks. She became sober three years later. Susan still comes in for monthly treatments to stay balanced and prevent any kind of relapse. If she's having a stressful time, such as the anniversary of her husband's passing, she comes in weekly.

Recap of Susan's Fire symptoms: panic attacks, insomnia, addiction, burning urination upon waking, menopause.

As you can now see, even the worst cases can see big improvement with just a few lifestyle tweaks. If you're feeling overwhelmed about your life or your mental or physical health, TCM can help. Also, remember to be gentle with yourself when going through something as challenging as a breakup or death of a loved one. Increase the number of Fire element–promoting foods in your diet (see lists at the beginning of this chapter), and you'll feel calmer and more carefree. A happy heart means a happy mind.

The secret of health for both mind and body is not to mourn for the past, not to worry about the future, or not to anticipate troubles, but to live the present moment wisely and earnestly.

—Siddhartha Gautama (The Buddha)

CHAPTER 9

Don't Worry, Be Happy

Stop Worrying and Overthinking

Recommended Foods

Foods to **nourish the Earth element** are some of my favorites: yams, garbanzo beans (hummus!), and squash. There are plenty of options from which to choose.

For a healthy spleen and stomach, eat these foods: millet, corn, carrots, cabbage, cauliflower, garbanzo beans, soybeans, squash, potatoes, string beans, yams, tofu, sweet potatoes, sweet rice, amaranth, peas, chestnuts, apricots, and cantaloupe.

Most people in Western cultures have some **spleen deficiency.** The causes are many, and just a few reasons include stress, too much computer use, overuse of antibiotics as medication and in nonorganic animal products, and a poor diet. Luckily, there are plenty of great-tasting foods to help nourish your spleen: oats, brown, red, or wild rice, spelt, squash, turnip, carrots, parsnips, black beans, peas, sweet potato, yam, pumpkin, garbanzo beans, leeks, ginger, garlic, fennel, black pepper, onion, nutmeg, and cinnamon.

Foods to Avoid or Minimize

It's best to avoid really rich or greasy foods, which are hard to digest when you have a weak spleen. You should also limit consumption of iced drinks, ice cream, seaweeds, raw veggies and fruit, dairy, sugar or sweetened foods, tofu, sprouts, and spinach. All of these examples are cold in nature, which compromises the strength of an already weak spleen. When it comes to raw fruits and vegetables, you can counteract the "cold" nature by adding ginger, garlic, or onion.

What? Me worry? Never.

Worry and overthinking are the two main emotions that affect the Earth element. And who hasn't spent a sleepless night because you haven't been able to turn off your brain? *What needs to get done tomorrow? What should have gotten done today? My boss is such a jerk. The kids are making me crazy.* The proliferation of smartphones and computers has made things even worse by keeping our minds turned on 24-7. There's almost no chance to escape it and tune out for a while. I'm guilty of it myself, and I know the consequences.

Every time you overthink, or spend too much time studying like I did when reviewing for my licensing exam, your spleen and stomach are weakened. Buddhists call it Monkey Mind. It means the mind is fluctuating, inconstant, or vacillating. The same thoughts keep going around and around in your mind, and you feel like it can't or won't stop. If you get upset that the wheels keep turning, it just makes it worse. Sound familiar? Even if you have a pretty easy life, quieting the mind can seem almost impossible.

Meditation and acupuncture are great tools for shutting down your Monkey Mind. Acupuncture is such a powerful tool that it can be used instead of anesthesia for surgery. It has been used during open-heart surgery in China for over forty years. That's how strong TCM is for calming the mind.

Your Earth element may also be compromised if you did not feel loved or nourished as a child, which was an issue for Terri, one of the case studies later in this chapter. This doesn't have to mean that what most of us would call actual abuse happened in childhood, just that you didn't feel loved or supported by your family, especially your parents. Maybe the parents worked a lot and weren't around, or just didn't say "I love you" very often (or at all). This type of upbringing can lead to the constant search for love and affection, which sometimes coexists with the attitude that one is undeserving of anyone's love and kindness.

The opposite situation—spoiling a child—can also have negative consequences, both emotionally and physically. The somatic ramifications are the same as not feeling loved, but the child's development can be stunted mentally in a very different way. Being overly mothered in childhood can manifest as a manipulative personality who whines to gain attention, complains constantly, has the feeling that no one really "gets" them, or distrusts people in general.

The Earth element is late summer, the color yellow, a sweet taste, dampness, transformation, and the organs are the stomach (yang) and spleen (yin). It's connected to blood vessels, patience, stability, and is a time to manifest and acknowledge the fruits of our labor (harvesting in late summer). Since it is at the center of the five elements, Earth is the most balanced between yin and yang. This element makes us capable of nurturing ourselves and those around us.

Worrying and overthinking are just two emotions that impact the spleen and stomach or manifest when they are weakened. There are actually several moods connected to them: obsessive thoughts, using your brain too much for work (like writing a book) or studying for school, the Monkey Mind, and being stuck in detrimental patterns, whether it be diet, relationships, work, or how you process your thoughts and feelings.

Being a yin organ, the spleen has a lot of responsibilities, both in Western and TCM terms. It's located below the stomach along the digestive tract and further aids in metabolism.

In the chart that follows, I've used a few strange terms when listing the spleen's Chinese functions. What do I mean by "keeps blood in vessels"? The spleen helps prevent bruising and varicose veins. Do you have bruises yet no clue where they came from? Does the discoloration last longer than it should? You may be prone to bruising or varicose or spider veins if you have a weak spleen.

Functions of the Spleen	
Western Medicine	**TCM**
Purifies the blood	Transforming food into nutrients
Stores and makes red blood cells	Moves qi throughout the body
Aids in healing injuries	Dries damp; lifts, pushes out stool
Supplies blood in heavy bleeding emergencies	Makes qi and blood, supports brain function, and keeps blood in vessels
	Stimulates small intestine function

What do I mean by "lifts"? Any kind of sagging or prolapse (drop of an organ), such as a hernia, prolapsed uterus, or premature sagging of skin, can be due to a weakened spleen. Sagging skin does come with age, of course, but some people's faces start drooping as early as in their twenties. Lifting can also be more figurative in meaning—such as lifting your spirits and energy levels. If you can't seem to get motivated or are always low energy, it can be the result of a fragile spleen. An example is Evan, who had sagging everything. He was forty when he first came in for treatment, but he looked fifty-five because of his sagging skin. He had two hernias and hemorrhoids that never seemed to go away. Evan's job as an engineer used a lot of brainpower, and he was also a worrywart. Even when things were going great for him, he thought about the worst possible outcome or wondered when the good would stop. He was never able to completely trust anyone or the potential for good things to come to fruition. He was also always bloated and gassy and had food sensitivities to about twenty foods, including dairy, gluten, pineapple, and shellfish. He also started having spider veins in his early twenties, which is considered quite young, especially for a man. Almost all his health issues were related to the spleen.

What do I mean by "dries damp"? The most obvious symptom is reducing water retention or edema. Dampness in TCM can also manifest as eczema, acne, foggy head or lack of concentration, excess weight, phlegm, forgetting dreams, mixing up words, cysts, fibroids, tumors, mucus, yeast infections, Candida, bladder infections, diarrhea, and an enlarged prostate. A healthy spleen would help dry the excess "damp" to reduce or clear these conditions.

One symptom to spotlight here is Candida. You may think that yeast is only a problem "down there," but it can affect the intestines and digestive tract as well. Candida can be hard to diagnose, because it shares symptoms with other health issues, such as irritable bowel syndrome and gluten intolerance. You might find yourself bouncing between doctors in an effort to find the true culprit of symptoms such as bloating, diarrhea, constipation, sinusitis, or headaches. If you answer "yes" to many of the questions below, you probably have Candida.

- Have you ever taken repeated or prolonged courses of antibiotics?

- Do you eat nonorganic animal products, which contain antibiotics and steroids?

- Have you taken a prolonged course of steroids or birth control pills?

- Have you been bothered by recurrent vaginal, prostate, or urinary tract infections?

- Are you bothered by hormone-related issues, including PMS, infertility, menstrual irregularities, or sexual dysfunction?

- Are you overly sensitive to certain odors?

- Do you have memory or concentration problems?

- Do you suffer from digestive issues?

- Does your skin itch, burn, or rash easily?

- Do some foods worsen your symptoms?

What next? Eliminate yeast-promoting foods. For a minimum of six weeks, eliminate foods that feed yeast and encourage its growth: sugar, dairy, yeast, fruit, grains, and fermented foods. Eat no more than 40 to 60 grams of carbohydrates a day. Focus on eating vegetables, nuts, seeds, and unprocessed oils, and drink plenty of water. The good news is that Candida is treatable with simple dietary changes and the right supplements. It can take a few months to really eliminate the yeast, so don't give up if your symptoms don't go away immediately. As the yeast starts to die off, you might feel sick. This is a really good sign, even though you don't feel well for a while. Die-off symptoms include nausea, acne, bloating, gas, yeast infections, headaches, muscle and joint soreness, change in bowel movements, fever or chills, abnormal sweating, sinus infections, fatigue, and dizziness. These manifestations will soon disappear. How you feel once the yeast is gone makes it totally worth it.

The spleen can affect several aspects of your health. Even though we can actually live without the spleen, being in charge of digestion and making qi means it's a pretty important organ.

Other symptoms of spleen deficiencies include irregular bowel movements—in most cases loose stools, but sometimes constipation (due to not having enough strength to push stool out)—fatigue after eating, gas, stomach pain, loss of appetite, nausea and vomiting, and food allergies and sensitivities. A spleen deficiency may also manifest with pain or temperature change along its channel, hemorrhoids, and varicose and spider veins, sugar cravings, pale and/or dry lips, anemia, fatigue, yellow complexion, and puffy eyes (especially under the eyes).

Craving sugar is probably the most common symptom I see in my clinic related to spleen deficiencies. It really does become a vicious cycle of eating it, feeling low, and wanting more. A majority of my patients are addicted to the white stuff. I have to highlight craving sugar again because so many people are hooked on it, sometimes without even realizing it. You don't have to drink two liters of soda a day or eat a batch of cookies in one sitting to be dependent on your daily dose(s) of the highly addictive white stuff. As you learned in chapter 7, sugar is hidden in a lot of foods. Make sure to read labels and look for these ingredients: barley malt, beet sugar, brown sugar, buttered syrup, cane juice crystals, cane sugar, caramel, carob syrup, caster sugar, confectioners' sugar, corn syrup, corn syrup solids, date sugar, demerara sugar, dextran, dextrose, diatase, diastatic malt, ethyl maltol, fructose, fruit juice, fruit juice concentrate, galactose, glucose, glucose solids, golden sugar, golden syrup, grape sugar, high fructose corn syrup, honey, icing sugar, invert sugar, lactose, malt syrup, maltodextrin, maltose, mannitol, maple syrup, molasses, muscovado sugar, panocha, raw sugar, refiner's syrup, rice syrup, sorbitol, sorghum syrup, sucrose, treacle, turbinado sugar, and yellow sugar. That's fifty names for sugar. Fifty. Only a culture obsessed with sweets would have so many options. Are you ready to just say "No!" to sugar? Remember, whatever you call it, it's still sugar.

Other spleen problems include excessive bleeding during menses, pale menstrual blood, and bleeding between periods; frontal/forehead headaches (usually with a dull ache); clouded thinking or mixing up words; slow metabolism or thyroid dysfunction; and weight gain, mainly in the belly.

As you can see, the health of your spleen is crucial to your general health. Without healthy digestion, nutrients can't be absorbed and used for energy, organ function, and immunity.

Functions of the Stomach	
Western Medicine	**TCM**
Stores food, aids digestion	Makes qi and fluids
Metabolizes nutrients and breaks down food into liquid	Metabolizes food and transports nutrients
Empties into small intestine	Regulates appetite
	Controls dissension of qi to small intestine

The stomach basically does what you would expect. Its functions are all related to digestion, but you may be unfamiliar with one phrase used in the chart above: "Controls dissension of qi to the small intestine." Basically, this means the stomach helps you poop. The stomach pushes digested food into the small intestine. If the health of the stomach is at all compromised, you may experience constipation.

The stomach is the organ most of us equate to digestion, and we would be correct. After the mouth and esophagus, our food goes into the stomach. We need a happy tummy to metabolize and absorb all those nutrient-rich foods. Like all yang organs, there are just a few symptoms related to an imbalanced stomach. A depleted stomach often shows up as nausea, vomiting, acid regurgitation, hunger without the desire to eat (nothing sounds good), excessive appetite, pain and temperature change along the channel, bloating, thirst, and hiccuping.

Overconsumption of food and drink has become all too common, leading to both stomach problems and weak spleens. If you tend to overeat, reducing your intake, even if it's vegetables, is the first step to a stronger spleen and digestion in general. Adding mood-boosting foods for the spleen and stomach will help even more.

CASE STUDIES

Terri

Let's go back to Terri, aged thirty-nine, who was diagnosed with hypothyroidism just before our first visit. She definitely did not feel warmth and support as a child, but it took several weeks before she opened up about it. I think a part of why she didn't want to talk about her parents and upbringing was because she felt wimpy for thinking her early years were at all challenging. She was never hit, always had a belly full of food, clean clothes, friends, and a roof over her head. Life wasn't bad, but it wasn't great either. Terri's dad was a workaholic. He wasn't mean to her, he just wasn't around. He missed holidays, some birthdays, and recitals at school. Terri felt like her dad didn't care about her. She doesn't remember him ever hugging her and showing any affection. Terri's mom, a housewife, was home much of the time, but she was usually busy with friends or organizing the next fundraiser for church. Terri's mom loved her sugar and would bake every day. Terri thought the sweet treats were her mom's way of showing love. It's no wonder that Terri developed an Earth imbalance at a young age and was addicted to sugar.

Terri did not want to go on the thyroid medication prescribed by her general practitioner due to her concerns about potential side effects. She also felt that drugs wouldn't permanently fix her thyroid, making her dependent on them the rest of her life. Her hypothyroid symptoms were a forty-pound weight gain in the last sixteen months, thinning hair, low energy (especially in the afternoon), feeling cold all the time, irregular menstrual cycle, and cracked skin on her heels.

Terri was also concerned about overeating, eczema, and pain along her inner calves and the spleen channel. Her skin condition made her very insecure, and she covered up with clothes as much as possible. She had been overweight as long as she could remember and had stayed about the same weight for almost eight years. But the forty-pound gain in just over a year was significant.

Her job as a computer analyst required constant brainpower. Terri was worried all the time. Although not diagnosed with OCD, her actions and mind-set were borderline obsessive. She was stuck in a pattern of constantly thinking about her problems but doing nothing to make changes in her life. She stayed in damaging romantic relationships out of insecurity, feeling unlovable, and thinking there was no way out. Her inability to be proactive was incredibly frustrating to her, a frustration that made her feel even more stuck.

Although she tended to overeat, Terri actually ate a pretty healthy diet, very California-style with lots of fresh organic produce. She ate a salad every day. She didn't eat any fast food or drink soda. But she was addicted to refined sugar and would eat large quantities of candy, chocolate, and cakes daily. Her need for sweets got to the point where she'd eat an entire cake in one sitting. Terri tried to give up her sweet treats, but couldn't. She eventually gave up even trying.

I focused on Terri's thyroid dysfunction, mental health, and sugar addiction. She came in for weekly treatments the first three months. She felt so great after that she was able to come in for monthly "tune-ups." I gave Terri very simple dietary suggestions and herbs to support her thyroid and spleen. She was tired of feeling tired and was willing to make lifestyle changes.

My suggestions for Terri included increasing her water intake, taking a multivitamin and an iodine supplement, and cutting out all refined sugar. Why more water? I actually have to encourage 95 percent of my patients to drink more water. (If you've forgotten why, take another look at chapter 7.) I also advised her to make sure all animal products she consumed were organic.

Addiction

When I see patients addicted to sugar, coffee, soda, or cigarettes, they must be ready to give up their addiction(s) before I can support them in this process. I let them decide whether or not going cold turkey or weaning slowly is best for them. When it comes to more serious addictions to drugs and alcohol, cold turkey seems to be the best way to go. With food addictions or eating disorders, and, of course, drugs and alcohol addiction, I recommend getting outside support—twelve-step programs, therapy, and rehab for drugs and alcohol. Having a strong support system is key in raising your chances of recovery. Sharing your commitment with others to give up whatever you're dependent on makes you more accountable to follow through with your decision.

Here's a sample of her meal plan.

Breakfast: oatmeal or hot quinoa cereal with berries.

Lunch: brown rice with black bean chili and pumpkin.

Snacks: juice with cabbage, carrots, pears, kale, ginger.

Dinner: quinoa topped with any steamed veggies, including bell pepper, cauliflower, and squash, a little tofu, ginger miso dressing, hemp seeds, sprouts, and nutritional yeast.

Terri was amazed by her improvements, and so was her endocrinologist. She lost fifteen pounds over three months. Her energy levels increased immediately, and her hair started to thicken within a month. Terri's eczema was also gone in just over a month—this made her just as happy as the weight loss—and she definitely worried less. Giving up sugar took a bit longer, but Terri was ready to say good-bye to oatmeal chocolate-chip cookies after about eight months of coming in to see me. She transitioned into a more carefree person and was able to start making decisions that benefited her and to be proactive in making positive changes. Her family and friends all commented on how much happier and laid-back she was. Terri still comes in for nutritional guidance, herbs, and treatment. She knows it helps her to keep stress levels to a minimum and stay on track with her eating habits.

Recap of Terri's Earth symptoms: obsessive worry, sugar cravings, hypothyroidism, weight gain, eczema, pain along spleen channel, fatigue.

Kristen

Now imagine a Type A personality with a weak spleen, an ambitious and high-strung overachiever and workaholic, always wanting to improve. All these traits compromise the Earth element. This was Kristen to a T.

Kristen was a fifty-five-year-old married mother of two who worked seventy hours a week in a very high-pressure job in a large multinational corporation. I see this trend of overworking more and more with my patients. Overwork and excessive stress from work is the norm, at least with the people I treat. They're so busy that oftentimes they don't even have an hour per month for a treatment.

Kristen's chief complaint was edema, or water retention, which she thought had been going on for eight months. She had it all over her body, including around her heart, which sometimes was very painful. Occasionally her feet and ankles swelled up, or her belly would look like she was five months pregnant. She started to have chest pain a few weeks before I first saw her. A stress test, a Holter monitor, and an electrocardiogram (ECG) all came back normal.

What is edema exactly? Edema occurs when capillaries leak fluid and the fluid builds up in surrounding tissues. You can sometimes reduce edema through changing lifestyle habits, like reducing your salt intake. Edema can be the result of sitting or staying in one position for too long, pregnancy, PMS, medications for pain, diabetes, beta-blockers, and estrogen imbalances. The more serious medical causes include kidney disease or failure, congestive heart failure, poor lymphatic drainage (usually from cancer surgery), varicose veins, or liver cirrhosis usually caused by alcoholism.

Kristen's doctor ruled out all of the possible causes for her edema and was stumped. Every test was done. She only drank alcohol a couple of times a month and didn't take any medication. She was postmenopausal, so no PMS. That's when Kristen called my office.

Mercury in Fish

Even the US Environmental Protection Agency (EPA) states nearly all seafood contains some mercury, although it says only pregnant women, nursing mothers, and young children need to be concerned. Mercury in seafood is the result of our streams and oceans becoming a dumping ground for pollution. The thought is the larger the fish and the higher up on the food chain, the higher the concentrations of mercury; some examples of these include shark, tuna, pike, marlin, and trout. Personally, I don't want *any* mercury in my body.

There are so many illnesses and conditions that have been linked to mercury poisoning. I won't list them all, but they include memory loss, insomnia, emotional instability, lupus, multiple sclerosis, hypothyroidism, unexplained elevated cholesterol, abnormal blood pressure (high or low), bleeding gums and loosened teeth, excessive salivation, burning sensation with tingling of lips or face, dizziness/vertigo, ringing in the ears, chronic headaches, allergies, fatigue, rashes, Bell's palsy, and muscle twitching.

So please think twice before eating that "healthy" tuna salad.

Kristen also complained of bruising very easily, gas and bloating, low back and shoulder pain when stressed (most of the time), and frontal (on her forehead) headaches, usually after meals. She was constantly thirsty, no matter how much water she drank. This was probably from her body's inability to properly absorb and excrete water.

With her high levels of stress and overwork, Kristen couldn't stop thinking or shut down her brain, especially at night. As a result, her spleen was very weak, and her sleep was poor. It was rarely restful, and even when on vacation, Kristen only slept five hours a night. She would have nightmares about missing important deadlines. Some of that was due to insomnia and some because of her work schedule.

Kristen ate one of the cleanest diets out of any of my patients. She had several food allergies and sensitivities, so she avoided most high allergen foods like dairy and gluten. She was a pescatarian (ate seafood rarely because of concern about mercury poisoning, but no meat) and ate plenty of organic vegetables and fruit daily.

Since her doctors were at a loss as to what to do for Kristen, I tested her for food allergies through a simple blood test done in my

Food Allergies

The incidence of food allergies is on the rise. Approximately fifteen million Americans suffer from food intolerance of some kind. According to the Centers for Disease Control and Prevention (CDC), food allergies among children rose 50 percent from 1997 to 2011. Those are some startling and scaring statistics. Mostly likely you or someone close to you suffers from some level of food sensitivity. Many of my patients come in for this very problem, but most don't realize allergies might be causing or contributing to other health issues.

Why is this increase occurring? I've found through research and my clinical experience that there are many different possible reasons. Among them are overconsumption of or too-early (under age six) exposure to high-allergen foods, genetically modified foods, side effects of certain vaccines, weakened immunity for those not exposed to high-allergen foods through breast milk, and overuse of antibiotics (either as medication or through nonorganic animal products).

Eight foods or groups of foods cause about 90 percent of all food allergies:

- Dairy products

- Eggs

- Shellfish (shrimp, crab, lobster)

- Fish (tuna, salmon, cod, halibut)

- Tree nuts (almonds, cashews, pecans, walnuts)

- Peanuts

- Soy

- Wheat/gluten

One of the tricky things about food allergies is that they don't always show up as you'd expect. Not everyone responds with an upset stomach, digestive complaints, or fatigue after eating. Unfortunately this is not something many doctors know, and they may be slow to diagnose.

Food allergy symptoms can be divided into categories. Digestive symptoms may include diarrhea, gas, abdominal pain, irritable bowel syndrome, ulcers, gallstones, leaky gut syndrome, celiac disease, weight gain, and vomiting. Emotional symptoms may include depression, ADD/ADHD, autism, panic attacks, and anxiety. Allergies may also manifest themselves on the skin as eczema, psoriasis, or rosacea. Signs of diminished immunity such as ear infections, asthma, chronic fatigue syndrome, or frequent flus/colds may also suggest an allergy issue. Allergies are even suspected as a cause of infertility, migraines/headaches, multiple sclerosis, and epilepsy.

If you have any of the above health concerns, please consult a qualified physician for diagnosis and treatment. There is hope! Healing or minimizing food allergies is now possible. Abstaining from those foods, acupuncture/acupressure, detoxification, proper nutrition, and appropriate supplementation are parts of the protocol. Boosting your immune system, cleansing your body of toxins, and healing any damage done to your digestive tract from the exposure to allergen foods will bring you optimal wellness. At a minimum, the result will most likely be a reduction in allergy symptoms, and at best a complete elimination of your allergies.

Treating food allergies requires some patience and dedication, but it's completely possible. A series of acupuncture treatments and temporary avoidance of the allergens are often key early steps in the healing process.

office. She was highly allergic to over thirty common foods. Some of these she knew about, because the allergic response was immediate and obvious. Almond butter on a piece of rice bread would immediately cause her to swell up and have bloating and gas. A glass of organic red wine would immediately result in a headache. But some of the results came as a surprise, such as sesame seeds, lentils, and blueberries (which were in her daily smoothie). Kristen had never felt sick after eating these foods.

Even with her hectic schedule, Kristen came to me twice a week for treatments the first two months, then weekly for three more months. She now has treatments every two weeks to make sure she stays healthy and keeps her stress to a minimum.

I put Kristen on a Chinese herbal formula to support her immune system, aid digestion, reduce stress, and reduce edema. I also had her take probiotics—healthy bacteria—daily. Probiotics are great for boosting the immune system and restoring the digestive tract to reduce food sensitivities and aid in digestion and metabolism of nutrients. Recent studies show that having enough healthy gut flora reduces anxiety, depression, and other mood disorders. Remember that if you get probiotics from a dairy source, they must be organic; if not, you're wasting your money. Nonorganic animal products have antibiotics and ste-roids in them that will cancel out the benefits of probiotics.

Since Kristen's diet in general was very clean and healthy, I only had to encourage her to eat more spleen-nourishing foods, eliminate seafood, and to avoid completely the foods she was allergic to while I treated the allergies. I also had her add lemon to her water to help with metabolism, detoxification, and water absorption.

Breakfast: juice made with celery, ginger, carrots, kale, romaine lettuce, beets, and pears.

Lunch: squash soup with ginger and steamed green beans, or split pea soup.

Snacks: veggie sticks (like turnips and celery), fresh cantaloupe and grapes or dried apricots and berries.

Dinner: baked sweet potato and a large salad with garbanzo beans, garlic, daikon radish sprouts, sunflower seeds, and peas.

Kristen's healing process took a few months, due to the severity of her symptoms and allergies. But she saw an almost immediate reduc-tion in her stress levels, and she was able to sleep restfully through the night within three weeks. She was also obviously much calmer after every treatment. The constant concern about work was almost gone. The edema was mostly gone after six months, but she is careful to prevent a relapse. Kristen gave up seafood after six months.

Recap of Kristen's Earth symptoms: edema, constant worrying, gas and bloating, frontal headaches, food allergies, shoulder tension, bruising.

There is a proliferation of weakened spleens in Western cultures. The way to a healthy spleen and stomach can take some lifestyle changes. Eating Earth-nourishing foods will give you more energy, contribute to weight loss, and help you shut down your brain a little more. If you find yourself obsessing about your day or the day to come, take the time to make yourself a soothing mug of ginger tea.

You cannot prevent the birds of sadness from passing over your head,
but you can prevent their making a nest in your hair.

—CHINESE PROVERB

CHAPTER 10

Heavy Metal: Grief and Sadness

Recommended Foods

Excess phlegm can accumulate in the lungs and/or sinuses. Runny nose, coughing up mucus, and sinus congestion or infection are all a result of phlegm in the lungs, but many foods can help: kelp, turnips, fennel, flaxseeds, cayenne pepper, watercress, garlic, ginger, mushrooms, and papaya. Definitely avoid dairy if you have any phlegm, as dairy is a form of mucus. Also stay away from peanuts and soy.

Lung qi deficiency can lead to shortness of breath, catching colds easily, fatigue, loss of voice, and excessive daytime sweating for no reason. To support the lung qi, eat these foods: rice, oats, carrots, mustard greens, sweet potatoes, yams, potatoes, fresh ginger, garlic, molasses, rice syrup, and barley malt.

When dry weather affects your lungs and breathing or aggravates your symptoms, you should include these foods into your daily routine: nori, almonds, pine nuts, peanuts, sesame seeds, soybeans, tofu, tempeh, soy milk, spinach, barley, millet, pear, apple, persimmon, barley malt, and rice syrup.

Heat in the lungs is a common problem in my clinic, especially in the winter. It manifests as coughing up green or yellow phlegm, a burning sensation when coughing, pneumonia, or bronchitis. Smokers always have excess heat in their lungs. Try these foods: cabbage, asparagus, bamboo shoots, banana, pears, oranges, lemon, watercress, cauliflower, apples, carrots, lime, bok choy, cantaloupe, apples, persimmons, papaya, peaches, strawberries, kelp, nori, figs, mushrooms, radish, Swiss chard, and pumpkin.

Make sure to avoid the following when you have heat in the lungs: ginger, onions, garlic, fennel, cinnamon, alcohol, and coffee.

Lung yin deficiency can manifest as a dry, hacking cough (that annoying cough that just won't go away, even after you're not sick anymore) and lung cancer. This is usually a chronic health complaint, but many foods can help: nori kombu, wakame, tofu, miso, pears, apples, oranges, bananas, peaches, strawberries, watermelons, tomatoes, string beans, persimmon, peanuts, and spirulina.

Any foods that are high in beta-carotene help protect the lungs' mucosal linings and defend them from illness. So make sure to eat some of these goodies on a daily basis: kale, sweet potato, carrots, spinach, turnip greens, collard greens, butternut squash, winter squash, romaine lettuce, cabbage, beet greens, coriander, basil, and parsley.

General support for the large intestine is needed for symptoms that include constipation, diarrhea, excessive thirst, polyps, hemorrhoids, gas, bloating, and loose stools. As with all yang organs, the large intestine has just a few foods to support it. Apart from fresh, high fiber foods in general, try these foods as well: tofu, black pepper, cabbage, corn, cucumber, eggplant, fig, lettuce, nutmeg, persimmon, rice bran, salt, spinach, basil, and white pepper.

Foods to Avoid or Minimize

For heat in the lungs: ginger, onions, garlic, fennel, cinnamon, alcohol, and coffee

For phlegm in the lungs: dairy, yeast, wheat, peanuts, soy, and sugar

When you have a cold: raw foods and dairy

Have you ever been so distraught over a death that you just couldn't recover? The tears just wouldn't stop, or possibly they never came at all. Or was it that great love you didn't want to say good-bye to, even years after the breakup? Or what about the time your best friend in high school hurt your feelings and you still can't seem to forgive and forget? You know it is detrimental to your health, but you still keep holding on to the memories.

We've all lost a loved one or close friend, whether through death or the end of a relationship. Sometimes grieving and letting go comes naturally. Really grieving a loss gets rid of people, habits, or things that are no longer serving us. But sometimes it gets stuffed down. Sometimes we can't say good-bye. We've all experienced the challenge of letting go of a relationship, a past hurt, or a harmful habit. These damaging habits can be physical, like eating junk food, or emotional, like staying in an abusive relationship. Sometimes we get so accustomed to feeling or acting a certain way that we don't realize what we're doing or that we're hurting ourselves and the people around us. How can we expect better if we hold onto the past?

Our Metal element and large intestine and lungs have to face some challenges and obstacles throughout our lives. Being sad, losing someone you love, being exposed to pollutants, catching a cold or bronchitis, and suffering from asthma all harm the Metal element. If it doesn't get enough attention, the lungs and/or large intestines will start to show signs of distress.

The Metal element is associated with fall, the color white, a pungent or spicy taste, dryness, the lungs and large intestines, and skin conditions. The lungs enable us to be inspired and welcome in new thoughts, ideas, and action steps. The large intestines eliminate all the junk, both physical and emotional. Someone with a prevalent Metal element will have a strong sense of self, but not in an egotistical way. This is simply someone who is sure of him- or herself. Someone with an imbalanced Metal element will go to the extreme of needing to do everything alone and not asking for help, but still wanting approval from everyone they know.

If you have any issues with your lung and/or large intestines, you most likely have a skin condition of some kind. Most skin disorders are the result of lung issues, but the large intestines can play a role as well. These issues can manifest as sensitive skin, rashes, hives, eczema, or acne. Acne can be the result of constipation. A buildup of toxins in our intestines will eventually make its way to the liver and get flushed out through the skin, thus causing acne.

As you've already learned, the emotions related to the Metal element are grief and letting go. They can also be sadness and possibly depression. Depression is usually a liver issue, but sometimes depression is the result of stuffing down one's grief for an extended period of time.

One client, Jerry, had lost his ten-year-old daughter in a fatal car accident. It had been five and a half years since she passed when he came to see me. Jerry just couldn't move on. Of course, you never completely get over the loss of a loved one, especially not your own child. But after a certain amount of time and grieving, most people start to feel at least some reprieve from the sadness. Jerry just couldn't. He barely slept. He woke up at 4:00 a.m. every morning and couldn't fall back asleep; he made his way through each day in a daze that never seemed to lift. He also developed hay fever and allergies to several pollens, a chronic cough from the postnasal drip, and itchy, red rashes on his right cheek that would come and go with seemingly no cause. Jerry's unresolved grief was making him physically ill. All of these symptoms stemmed from his depleted Metal element.

We know the lungs are doing our breathing for us. Unless you meditate, have asthma, or do a lot of yoga, you might not be paying much attention to your breathing, at least not until you catch a cold or bronchitis.

Functions of the Lungs	
Western Functions	**Chinese Functions**
Taking in oxygen	In charge of the immune system
Respiration	Assists spleen in sending qi to the heart to make and move blood
	Opens to the nose for sense of smell
	Descends qi to help large intestines push out stool
	Descends qi to aid bladder in pushing out urine

In the chart on the previous page, some strange concepts are listed in the Chinese functions of the lungs. "Pushing out urine and stool" seems to make no sense, right? The lungs aren't physically connected to the bladder or intestines in any way, at least not in our Western thinking. As you already learned earlier in the chapter, the large intestines are the other half of the Metal element. But helping with urination is a strange concept. In Chinese medicine the lung and large intestine interact with each other to rid the body of toxins even though they're not connected in any way we can see with our eyes. Urination was difficult for Jerry because his weak lungs could not help push it out.

"Assists the spleen in sending qi to the heart to make and move blood" is the function I find most fascinating. Western medicine was a little late in figuring this one out. This idea of the lung and heart connection wasn't "discovered" in the West until the thirteenth century, but the Chinese knew centuries earlier that the lungs send oxygen to the heart. The spleen, with the help of the lungs, sends blood and qi to the heart to help it pump blood.

"Opens to the nose" refers to the lungs' role in controlling our breathing, but also to their influence on our sense of smell. That's where the reference "opens to the nose" comes in. Anyone who has had a cold can remember not being able to smell or taste a thing. Jerry lost his sense of smell due to his recent development of allergies. He couldn't take deep breaths or smell the roses.

The symptoms of the imbalanced lungs are mostly related to our physical lungs. We undeniably can't live without them. They include allergies (mostly environmental, but sometimes food allergies, too), frequent colds/illnesses, shortness of breath on exhale, asthma, constipation or loose stools, weak immunity, skin conditions (eczema, rosacea, psoriasis, acne, dermatitis, hyperkeratosis, dry or oily skin), pain or temperature change or injury along the channel, affected sense of smell, bronchitis, pneumonia, nasal congestion, sinusitis, craving spicy foods, and cold hands.

The large intestine is the other key organ to consider when treating grief, sadness, and the ability to let go. The large intestine helps us to let go of what is toxic to us mentally and physically. Most people know that the large intestine is in charge of bowel movements, but it really does so much more. It even has an influence on our state of mind.

Functions of the Large Intestine	
Western Medicine	**TCM**
Metabolizes nutrients	Removes waste
Removes waste from the body	Receives fluids from small intestine
Absorbs water	Letting go of emotional waste
Contains lymph nodes for immunity	

You might not even realize that the intestines contain lymph nodes that are vital to your immunity. Before taking anatomy and physiology, I always thought lymph nodes were in the neck and armpits, but they're really all over the body. We have between five hundred and seven hundred of them located from our sinuses down to our knees. Lymph nodes are located in the spleen, throat, thymus gland, and along the spine. The large intestines also contribute to our immune system by providing healthy bacteria. These good bacteria also benefit your state of mind by influencing your brain chemistry.

Symptoms of imbalanced large intestines include constipation or loose stools, diarrhea, difficulty letting go, pain or temperature change along the channel, acne, sensitive skin, pain in the intestines, and abdominal distention or pain. Tennis elbow is one large intestine–related ailment I'd like to highlight. Tennis elbow hurts along the large intestine channel at the elbow. All my patients suffering from tennis elbow also experience constipation. The question can be asked, does the tennis elbow cause the constipation, or does the constipation predispose you to injuring your elbow? Usually the answer is obvious in each case: Either the injured person was constipated for years before the elbow stared to hurt, or constipation occurred after the injury. Chinese medicine believes that when an element or organ suffers an imbalance or weakness, the person will be predisposed to injury or pain along the channel related to that organ. This might sound outrageous or totally absurd, but I see this coincidence almost daily in my clinic.

Bowel Movements

If one's bowels move, one is happy; and if they don't move, one is unhappy. That is all there is to it.
—Lin Yutang, 1937

Bowel movements are an invaluable way to help figure out what's going on with your insides. Yes, I know. Who wants to talk about those? My younger (and sometimes older) patients always giggle when I ask about their poop. Having one to three healthy, pain-free movements a day is key to your overall health. Getting rid of waste and toxins is vital. If they are loose, dry, appear several times a day, or not daily (without coffee!), you could have a problem. In Western terms, bowel issues can be caused by any of the following: low-fiber diet, stress, food allergies, irritable bowel syndrome, Crohn's disease, leaky gut syndrome, lack of healthy fats (more on those later), dehydration, side effects from certain medications, parasites, anemia, or Candida.

If your poop isn't great, it could definitely have an impact on your general health. The buildup of stool can lead to fatigue, weight gain, mood swings, insomnia, compromised immunity, and overgrowth of bad bacteria.

Difficulty letting go is the emotion related to the large intestine. Susan, whom you met in chapter 8, is a good example of the connection between the large intestine and grief/letting go. She was severely constipated after her husband's death. She would only go once a week, or even less often. Susan said she'd been this way since she was a kid, but the constipation worsened after her husband's death. She eventually realized she'd always had a hard time letting go physically and emotionally, even as a child. Susan grew up in an alcoholic and abusive home. She was too terrified to ever relax and was always on guard. Susan said that any time she would start to relax, her mom and older siblings could sense her vulnerability and attack her. Many therapists would agree that abused children hold on to their stools because it's the only thing they can control. Unfortunately, Susan kept this pattern into her adulthood. She became regular within a few weeks of her treatments.

Leaky gut is one of the more severe indications of an imbalanced large intestine. Sounds pretty gross, doesn't it? Well it is. And it's just what it sounds like, too. The intestines become permeable, allowing toxins, bacteria, viruses, fungi, and parasites to enter the blood. Ewww! The microvilli in the large intestine are damaged and are unable to produce crucial enzymes needed for the absorption of nutrients. Leaky gut can cause a whole host of health issues, usually misdiagnosed and mistreated. These include digestive complaints, such as gas, constipation, and/or diarrhea, chronic fatigue syndrome, skin conditions, fuzzy thinking, mood swings, weakened immunity, chronic joint or muscle aches, asthma, bronchitis, respiratory infections, sinus congestion, and food allergies.

The causes of leaky gut include gluten intolerance and food sensitivities; overuse of antacids, antibiotics, and nonsteroidal anti-inflammatory drugs (NSAIDs) such as ibuprofen, aspirin, or naproxen; smoking; overconsumption of alcohol; parasites; Candida; and overeating regularly.

To heal a leaky gut, you should temporarily eliminate all of the following:

- Dairy

- Junk and processed foods

- Refined grains, especially white flours

- Legumes

- Starchy vegetables—beets, carrots, potatoes, pumpkin, turnips, yams

- High-glycemic fruits—bananas, dried fruits, fruit juices

- Refined and fake sugars

- Alcohol, sodas, and caffeinated drinks

To help heal a leaky gut, eat as much organic food as you can, add lemon to your water daily, and try any of the following foods: nonstarchy vegetables, including alfalfa sprouts, artichokes, asparagus, bean sprouts, beet greens, bell peppers, bok choy, broccoli, brussels sprouts, cabbage, cauliflower, celery, chives, cilantro, collard greens, cucumber, dandelion greens, eggplant, endive, escarole, fennel, garlic, ginger, green beans, horseradish, kale, leeks, okra, onions, radishes, romaine lettuce, mustard greens, parsley, pickles, sauerkraut, scallions, snap peas, snow peas, spaghetti squash, spinach, summer squash, swiss chard, tomatoes, watercress, and zucchini. Also eat fresh fruits, including apples, apricots, berries, cantaloupe, cherries, currants, dates, figs, grapefruit, grapes, honeydew melon, kiwi, limes, mangoes, nectarines, oranges, papaya, peaches, pears, persimmons, pineapple, plums, pomegranates, tangerines, and watermelon.

I also recommend taking supplements such as digestive enzymes, probiotics, Chinese herbs, L-glutamine, omega-3 supplements from plant sources, and multivitamins.

There is hope! The microvilli in the small intestine can be repaired. They normally regenerate within four to five days. The healing process may take longer, depending on the severity of the damage.

CASE STUDIES

Samuel

Samuel was a sweet, shy boy. He was a small eleven-year-old who had lived with severe asthma since he was an infant. Samuel's mother brought him to see me in hopes of reducing his symptoms and medications. I see a lot of patients with asthma, but Samuel had a pretty serious case of it. His small stature was most likely due to the medications/steroids he had taken for the asthma most of his life. He couldn't partake in sports and had been hospitalized four times already. He wanted so badly to run and play and get into trouble with all the other boys, but even on medication, he was short of breath most of the time. With his asthma, he was prone to bronchitis and pneumonia, so he took antibiotics an average of three times a year. With even the hint of a chest cold his doctor put him on medication so he could still breathe.

Samuel also suffered from eczema, which is common among asthma sufferers. He had it on his scalp, elbows, and knees. It was always there, but it flared up when he was sick and made him insecure. Samuel would sweat without any exertion, which particularly embarrassed him in school. He also experienced gas and bloating after most meals. Samuel said his tummy hurt most of the time. He was sensitive and easily moved to tears. He told me he often felt anxious, especially around other children. He was often teased about his height and inability to compete in sports.

Samuel ate healthier than the average American boy: No SAD diet for him. His mom bought almost all organic produce and animal products. Unfortunately, he had sweets several times per day, including sweetened cereal, sweetened "juice," and dessert after dinner. He also consumed dairy at almost every meal. This was important for me to know, as dairy and sugar are the first two things I always suggest giving up for anyone suffering from asthma and/or eczema. They deplete the immune system and cause inflammation and phlegm to build up.

Samuel's asthma, even with medication, woke him up several nights per week. He also had bad dreams most nights, which also woke him and left him agitated. He often dreamed that he was choking and crying and sometimes awoke doing both.

I treated Samuel with acupressure, an excellent alternative to acupuncture for children (or anyone) afraid of needles. Acupressure is the exact same healing concept as acupuncture except that slight pressure with a finger is used on acupoints instead of acupuncture needles. I also gave him a multivitamin for children and a special Chinese herbal formula focused on his asthma.

Changing Samuel's diet was key to alleviating his asthma. Nine times out of ten, when asthmatics eliminate dairy and sugar (refined, not including fresh fruit), they feel better within a few weeks. I also recommended several of the foods that support the Metal element. He was ready to give up most sweets once I told him he'd start breathing better, though his evening ice cream was the hardest for him. Here's a sample meal plan I used to treat Samuel:

Breakfast: unsweetened almond milk smoothie with apples, pears, strawberries, and cantaloupe, or quinoa hot cereal (similar to oatmeal) with cinnamon and bananas.

Lunch: sandwich on gluten-free bread with tofu salad, watercress, Vegenaise, mustard, sprouts, Daiya cheese, pickles.

Snacks: fruit salad including peaches, pears, and blueberries, or hummus and carrot sticks.

Dinner: sushi with seaweed, brown rice, sesame seeds, spinach, and avocado, and fresh ginger and miso soup.

Improving your eating habits is difficult at any age. But children can definitely be very stubborn. When I explained to Samuel that eating these foods would help him breathe, he was highly motivated. Having your child become a part of the cooking process and making it fun and exciting to eat fruits and vegetables can help a lot. Give your meals creative names to make them giggle. Also, hiding veggies is a great trick. Spinach and carrots mixed in with a fruit smoothie will get past even the pickiest of eaters. It's best to avoid rewarding children with sugar, because it will encourage your child to want unwholesome foods.

Samuel's eczema was gone within a month of getting rid of dairy and sugar. His asthma showed marked improvement after just three treatments. Samuel was able to reduce his medications within a month. After six months, he was completely off all medication, though he did keep an inhaler on hand just in case. Samuel joined his local baseball team and had never been happier. Since he was no longer taking steroids for his asthma, he had a big growth spurt: three inches in eight months. Emotionally, Samuel became much more confident and less anxious, and started sleeping through the night after just two months. He came in less often as his condition improved, and once he was better, he came in only for monthly maintenance.

Recap of Metal symptoms for Samuel: asthma, eczema, gas, crying in sleep, themes in dreams.

Mark

Talk about being blocked up. Mark had problems going to the bathroom for literally decades. He was sixty-eight years old, divorced, retired, and had three adult children. His chief complaint was constipation since childhood. Mark was always gassy and bloated, because of the buildup of stool in his intestines. Laxatives and enemas helped him go at most once a week. Without them, he could go two weeks with nothing happening. How painful does that sound?

Mark was in pretty good shape, especially considering his history of excessive drug use, including methamphetamines, alcohol, marijuana, and LSD. He now only occasionally drank alcohol in small amounts. He stopped taking all drugs about ten years before coming to see me.

His only other health issues were pain along the large intestine channel in both arms, hip pain, and impotence. He took Viagra; even though it caused heart palpitations, he adamantly refused to stop taking it.

Mark had a lot of pent-up emotions. He had a really hard time letting go of past hurts and disappointments, especially his own mistakes. He also admitted that he had only cried once since giving up drugs. Mark was a victim of sexual and physical abuse as a child. Years of therapy only put a dent in the pain he held onto.

Mark slept through the night but had a troubling, recurring dream a few nights a week. This nightmare had been with him since the abuse started, at about age five. He said there was always a scaly male monster covered in boils trying to hurt him. Whenever he had this dream, Mark would wake up very tense, sometimes choking and unable to breathe.

Mark had a great California diet—plenty of fresh fruits and vegetables, all organic and locally grown. Mark drank two to three liters of water per day and ate only whole grains and some nuts and seeds. He got plenty of fiber and healthy fat to aid in digestion, so being constipated made no sense from a Western perspective. He had sought help from his doctor (who didn't ask a single question about his diet), and regular colonoscopies showed no structural problems.

Whenever one of my patients has similar digestion problems and eats a wholesome diet, I immediately assume it's the result of his or her emotional state. We did emotional release treatments along with supporting the intestines for the first month of weekly sessions.

Mark is one of a very few of my patients who didn't need many dietary changes. We did test for food allergies, because this can cause digestive upset; he tested negative for any food sensitivities. He was also given an herbal formula to address all his complaints. I did recommend foods that support the intestines from a Chinese nutritional perspective, as exemplified in the following meal plan:

Breakfast: grapefruit and gluten-free toast with nut butter, topped with banana.

Lunch: baked yam, steamed broccoli, and spinach and mustard greens over wild rice.

Snacks: peppermint tea, olive and eggplant spreads on rice crackers, prunes.

Dinner: corn chowder and a salad with cabbage, cucumber, spinach, and figs.

On his second visit, Mark came in with a big smile on his face. He had gone to the bathroom five days out of seven. He hadn't used a laxative once. He also had the very cathartic experience of crying for most of the weekend after two treatments. After six weeks, he was going to the bathroom at least once a day. Mark said he never felt better. His impotence also gradually went away, and he was able to stop taking Viagra after four months. The pain in Mark's arms and hips was gone almost immediately.

Recap of Metal symptoms for Mark: constipation, themes in dreams, difficulty with grief and letting go, inability to cry.

Patricia

I'd like to share another constipation story that was connected to a patient's mental state. This is to emphasize how much your emotions impact your physical health. Any issues involving bowel movements can be symptoms of difficulty letting go of the past or unresolved grief.

A healthy twenty-eight-year-old female named Patricia came to me with severe constipation (going only once every ten days for almost two years) as her chief complaint. Before that she had been going to the bathroom daily. She ate a healthy diet filled with fiber and fresh produce. Patricia also drank plenty of water. Every medical test you can think of had been done. I asked one simple question that gave me the answer I needed. "Did anything upsetting or traumatic happen when you first started experiencing constipation?" Her face lit up and she immediately said she had gone through a very painful breakup with her boyfriend and still wasn't over him. Ta-da!

Fiber: It Does the Body Good

Did you know that we're supposed to get at least 30 grams of fiber a day? The average American, however, eats only 15 grams per day. No wonder everyone is bloated, irregular, and at high risk for heart disease. And if you don't poop, your body reabsorbs toxins it's trying to flush out. One of the results: Colon cancer is now the third leading cause of cancer-related death in the United States.

Keep in mind that fiber is found only in plant foods and never in animal products. No wonder those who consume the Standard American Diet are clogged up. We're supposed to go three times a day. I can tell you most of my patients are lucky if they have a bowel movement once a day. I've seen some cases of once every ten days!

Benefits of Fiber

- Prevents colon cancer, constipation, colitis, hemorrhoids, gallstones, and varicose veins.

- Lowers cholesterol and helps prevent and manage diabetes.

- Slows the absorption of food, thus reducing blood glucose levels and increasing weight loss.

- Removes heavy metals and toxins and reduces the side effects of radiation.

Some Sources of Fiber

Fruits and vegetables (1 medium size, unless otherwise noted)

Apple with skin	3.0 grams
Banana	2.0 grams
Pear with skin	4.5 grams
Orange	2.0 grams
Prunes	3.0 grams
½ cup brussels sprouts	4.5 grams
1 large carrot	2.9 grams
½ cup broccoli	2.7 grams
Potato with skin	4.0 grams
½ cup corn	1.5 grams

Legumes, grains, nuts, and seeds (½ cup)

Barley	4.0 grams
Black beans	5.5 grams
Brown rice	1.5 grams
Garbanzo beans	6.0 grams
Green peas	6.9 grams
Kidney beans	6.5 grams
Lentils	4.5 grams
Lima beans	6.5 grams
Oats	3.0 grams
Pinto beans	5.9 grams

Tips

As you increase your fiber intake, pay attention to your use of medications and certain minerals (particularly calcium, iron, and zinc). You may need to adjust your medications, especially insulin. If you take a fiber supplement, never take your medications or supplements at the same time. Your body could take a little while to adjust to getting the fiber it needs, so you might be a bit gassy at first; this will pass. Drinking plenty of water and chewing on fennel seed will reduce the toots. See how important it is to get enough fiber? And how easy it is? Stock up on hummus, carrot sticks, and split pea soup, and you'll be good to go. No pun intended.

I gave her an acupuncture treatment and some herbs to help with the difficulty letting go of her ex. Patricia was regular within a few days without any laxatives or colonics. She also felt like she had finally said good-bye.

Just to make sure Patricia stayed healthy, I suggested foods to support and maintain her healing process.

Breakfast: raw almond butter on rye toast and juice with pears, beets, kale, ginger, carrots, and cucumber.

Lunch: burrito with avocado, kidney beans, wild rice, and salsa.

Snacks: whole grain or rice crackers spread with pumpkin seed "pâté," dried fruit and almonds, and bananas.

Dinner: brown rice noodles with tomato sauce and cannellini beans topped with pine nuts.

It's really easy to incorporate lung-nourishing foods into your daily regimen (see the list at the beginning of the chapter). I recommend eating some of them regularly, even if you don't have any obvious lung issues. You can easily support your Metal element by eating them. Don't let things get out of hand like Mark and Patricia did. Shore up your immune system, and you won't get stopped up or sick nearly as much.

To nurture one's life and health is mainly accomplished by cultivating one's mind. If the mind is calm and clear, the spirit is in a pure and healthy world, if the spirit is in a healthy world, how can the illness enter you?

—A COLLECTION OF EFFECTIVE PRESCRIPTIONS
BY LIANG WEN KE, QING DYNASTY

CHAPTER 11

Afraid of the Big, Bad Wolf: Anxiety

Recommended Foods

In this fast-paced world, the kidneys are constantly taking a beating. So it's a good idea to eat the following foods, whether you're displacing any symptoms of **general kidney weakness** or not: grapes, plums, boysenberries, celery, turnips, watercress, asparagus, millet, endive, cabbage, black beans, amaranth, rye, barley, quinoa, oats, kelp, nori, chlorella, miso, tangerines, plums, cinnamon, dill seed, and chives.

Kidney yin deficiency can manifest in any of these symptoms: insomnia, night sweats, anxiety, dryness, and fear. Increase your intake of the following foods to increase the yin of your kidneys: beets, carrots, yams, chlorella, kelp, spirulina, black sesame seeds, radish, sweet potatoes, mung beans, kidney beans, black beans, soybeans, string beans, watermelon, blueberries, blackberries, and aloe vera gel.

Kidney yang deficiency may cause you to experience low back pain, coldness, and diarrhea, with many symptoms worse in the morning. Dig into these foods to increase your yang: walnuts, black beans, quinoa, ginger, cloves, cinnamon, leeks, fennel, and anise.

Foods to Avoid or Minimize

For **kidney yang deficiency:** raw foods, iced drinks, and minimize fruit.

Did you know that forty million people will experience high levels of anxiety in the United States this year? Damn, that's a lot of people. No wonder the number of people taking antianxiety medications has gone up 30 percent in the last ten years. Do these medications really fix the underlying cause of anxiety? The answer for most is a resounding "No!" The primary symptoms are just masked for as long as you're taking the medication. Not only is the problem still there, but the unresolved issues can make you physically ill as well.

Ask anyone who's experienced it: Anxiety and panic attacks suck. Luckily, TCM is great for treating and healing why you have them in the first place. Who wants to go through life on edge or fearful all the time, or afraid that you're going to have a panic attack, causing more anxiety? There is a way to heal them once and for all.

Melanie, age forty-four, was of those unlucky people who had been suffering from anxiety and depression since high school. She had been taking some form of anti-anxiety medication and/or anti-depressants for twenty years before she came to my clinic for treatment. Melanie said she couldn't function or sleep without them, and whenever she tried stopping them (with her doctor's help), the anxiety would come back. She still had a low-grade fear even with the medication, and her depression never really lifted. Almost every time a new drug came on the market, her psychiatrist would switch her prescription. Sometimes they worked; sometimes they didn't. She came to me because she was ready to get off the roller-coaster ride. Initially, Melanie's fear protected her from her abusive stepfather. As an adult, anxiety and fear were controlling her life.

Fear can be a good thing. I realize I might sound crazy for saying this, but think about it: Fear gets you out of bad predicaments or helps you to avoid dangerous situations. Remember the last time you were cut off on the freeway? Your response was pretty quick, and you avoided an accident. Fear is what helped you to safety.

Unfortunately, most people I treat and know feel some level of anxiety or fear on a regular basis. They're so used to the anxiety that they just assume it's a part of being alive; being anxious is fundamental to who they are. All of them say they'd love to feel this way less often and less intensely, but they don't see a way out.

Taking care of the kidneys is crucial for optimal health. The kidneys are the source of yin and yang and our vital essence. If they're at all compromised, the rest of our organs will be sickly as well. If the kidneys are run-down, the healing process is much slower. Unfortunately, modern living is taking its toll on almost everyone's kidneys. What weakens the kidneys? Overwork, exposure to toxins, eating too much animal protein, stress, excessive intake of alcohol, drugs and many medications, and poor sleeping habits are some of the key culprits. See what I mean? Who doesn't experience at least one of these on a regular basis?

The kidneys and bladder are associated with the Water element. Water is connected to winter, its associated taste is salty, and it is thought to open to the ears, bones, and hair. Water is the most yin of the elements, and winter is the most yin time of year. It is a time of rest, reflection, meditation, looking inward, staying inside, rejuvenation, and contemplation. A person with a strong Water element is bright, flexible, and soft without being weak. They will be smart with their time, money, energy reserves, never overdoing it or being stingy with their talents. An imbalanced Water element may manifest as having difficulty keeping to decisions or being fully committed.

"Opens to the ears" means that the kidney's health is directly connected to your hearing. If you have hearing loss, sensitivity, deafness, or high-pitched ringing in the ears, you could have a Water imbalance of some kind. If you experience ringing in the ears, however, make sure to check that it isn't a structural issue or damage to your eardrums.

The Water element influences bones and hair as well. Weakened kidneys may show as dull, thin, or brittle hair. The aging process slowly weakens the Water element, leading to osteoporosis or arthritis in many of the elderly. When a child or young adult is afflicted with arthritis, their kidneys mostly likely have been severely damaged.

Functions of the Kidneys	
Western Medicine	**TCM**
Filter blood and urine (separate waste products from the blood that will go out with your urine)	Urination, reproduction, growth, supports organ function
Conserve water, salts, and electrolytes	Pull diaphragm down to aid in inhaling
Regulate blood pressure	Main source of yin and yang

The kidneys are in charge of producing and storing yin, yang, and source qi. This means that if your kidneys are weak and depleted of yin and/or yang, you will probably have deficiencies throughout your organs.

In Chinese medicine, your adrenal glands are actually considered the same organs as your kidneys. There's no distinction between the two, so I want to spend a little time on them. Your adrenals are two small glands that sit on top of your kidneys and help create energy. They regulate your stress response and secrete hormones, including aldosterone. When they've been overtaxed, they become fatigued, leading to the following symptoms: chronic fatigue, insomnia, being easily overwhelmed, craving salty and/or sweet foods, sensitivity to light or cold, difficulty concentrating, poor digestion, irritable bowel syndrome, frequent colds, PMS- and menopause-related problems, low blood pressure, allergies, arthritis, low libido, anxiety, panic attacks, and depression.

You'll see there is some overlap with kidney symptoms. Any of these symptoms sound familiar? If so, the foods I recommend for the kidneys should help alleviate adrenal fatigue and its symptoms as well. The modern lifestyle I mentioned earlier contributes to the weakening of your adrenals.

The purpose of the bladder is the same in both Western and Chinese functions. It collects urine from your kidneys and stores it until it is full enough to empty. This process of urination is to eliminate waste.

Since the kidneys play such an important role in our general health in TCM, their imbalance can manifest in dozens of ways. Patients who come to me for anxiety are always amazed when I ask if they have any of the following symptoms. It's not because I'm a mind reader; it's because their anxiety contributed to their ailments or vice versa. Just as the function of the bladder is pretty simple, so are its TCM symptoms. They include any urinary issues or infections, bed-wetting, incontinence, occipital (base of the skull) headaches, and pain or temperature change along its channel, as well as the following:

- Low back/knee pain and weakness, high-pitched tinnitus/ears ringing, hearing loss, genetic diseases, impotence, infertility, insomnia, hair loss, excessive or lack of sex appetite, premature graying and aging, arthritis, weak bones/osteoporosis, craving salt, and poor short-term memory.

- Congenital disorders: developmental disability, slow learning, delayed development, and intellectual disability.

- Emotional problems such as panic attacks, mental illness, phobias, anxiety, and emotional instability.

Given how the modern lifestyle negatively affects the kidneys, it makes sense that almost every person I see has some kidney symptoms. Wendy and Dawn were two of my more complex cases, with a whole host of health issues related to their fear and anxiety.

CASE STUDIES

Wendy

One patient who will always be close to my heart is Wendy. When she first came to see me, Wendy was forty-two years old, single, and worked part time from home. She initially came in for pain along the bladder channel—along her hamstrings, low back, and knees. When she first arrived, I immediately noticed very dark circles under her eyes and her thinning hair. She was also incredibly shy and nervous.

Wendy didn't know acupuncture and TCM could help with anything apart from pain, so she didn't mention most of her other health issues in her paperwork. I had to gently draw her out of her shell to learn of other physical ailments, most of which were related to her anxiety: a weak bladder, insomnia, dry mouth, nightmares, constipation, and environmental allergies. She had a history of very heavy periods, for which she was taking the birth control pill to regulate her cycle.

Wendy had a history of physical, emotional, and sexual abuse, which led to her mental health issues. She was also a recovering anorexic and bulimic. She was diagnosed as a paranoid schizophrenic after a psychotic break in 1996 and was taking several medications, including Prozac, risperidone, Wellbutrin, Paxil, and Zoloft.

Wendy was greatly affected by her traumatic history, which anyone would be. She had a lot of anxiety and fear, low self-esteem, and difficulty dealing with any change outside of her routine. She had difficulty keeping to commitments and would often slack off on obligations. Due to her lack of trust in other people, she had only a couple of friends and a job that could be done at home. She worried a lot, feared people would not like her or would be mean, and was constantly afraid of men taking advantage of her. Even with all this, Wendy was hopeful about her future and wanted to improve her health and the quality of her life. I was really impressed (and still am) by her bravery and determination to face her fears.

Wendy had been taking medication to help her sleep for almost twenty years. She never tried to go without it, because it was thought that lack of sleep could trigger another psychotic episode (and I fully agreed). Even with sleeping pills and a solid eight hours of sleep, Wendy normally woke up tired. This may have been partly due to a side effect of her medications.

Because she came in looking very depleted and pale, I suspected she had anemia and elevated liver enzymes. I immediately sent her in for blood work to check due to her long history of medications. My suspicions were right on target. Like most people with a history of eating disorders, she was anemic. Wendy's digestive tract was unable to absorb nutrients because of the use of diet pills, laxatives, and binging and purging. The anemia affected her energy levels, and it also played a part in her mood and tight muscles. Because her liver enzymes were also elevated, I normally would suggest a five-day liver cleanse, which reduces solid food intake for a few days, but you still get all the nutrients you need through soups and smoothies. I knew this wouldn't be a viable option for Wendy given her eating disorder history. So I just incorporated some options into her meal plan, including some liver-supporting herbs in her formula and some foods that naturally clean out toxins.

Along with acupuncture and food suggestions, I created a very simple Chinese herbal formula and prescribed some supplements, including probiotics (healthy bacteria for digestion and immunity), digestive enzymes, iron, and a vitamin B complex.

I asked Wendy to eat iron sources that were easy to digest, including pumpkin seeds, chard, broccoli, lentils, and tofu. She started eating many of the foods that nourish the kidneys and flush the liver of toxins. Also with Wendy's history, absorption of nutrients from some foods was a challenge. Since she was found to be anemic, many of her doctors then insisted she had to eat beef several times per week. Wendy said she felt sick after eating the beef and was constipated for a few days, but she felt pressured into eating it once a week. Being told she had to do something she was uncomfortable doing, especially in relation to food, triggered a major anxiety episode. Luckily Wendy recovered pretty quickly and learned some alternative and better sources of iron.

I talked extensively with Wendy about what would be a realistic meal plan for her. I wanted to make sure she felt comfortable with one that she would actually follow through on. Wendy had to be an active participant in her healing for it to really work. Again, these foods were created specifically for Wendy, but they can help anyone with similar issues.

Breakfast: tofu scramble with ginger, yellow curry, spinach, shredded carrots, and squash.

Lunch: sushi with seaweed, brown rice, avocado, daikon radish, black sesame seeds, ginger, and miso soup.

Snacks: watermelon, plums, blackberries, boysenberries, blueberries, grapes.

Dinner: baked purple potato, steamed asparagus and string beans, and millet with black beans.

After just a few short weeks, Wendy's progress was pretty incredible. Her long-term goals were a bit slower to be realized than some patients, because as I wrote earlier, I was very careful not to overwhelm her with changes. A few years later, she is now in less physical pain, with only occasional muscle tightness. Wendy has a healthy level of self-esteem and is able to speak up for herself, is less shy, has a fulfilling job, and has made some new friends. She was able to reduce the dosages of a few medications and only rarely takes a sleeping pill. (Wendy stopped taking the pill after two years with no negative consequences.) She still sees me for monthly tune-ups and is feeling great.

Recap of Wendy's Water-related symptoms: pain along her hamstrings, insomnia, mental illness, dry mouth, weak bladder, dark circles under the eyes.

Dawn

Panic attacks are more common than you might think. About 3 percent of the US population (six million people) experience them. Women are twice as likely to be afflicted with them as men. Panic attacks can so debilitating as to drastically reduce one's quality of life. Poor Dawn was one of those people.

When I met her, Dawn was a married, thirty-eight-year-old mother of two with a full-time job. She had started having panic attacks about two years before coming to see me, sometimes as often as three times per week. Despite taking Xanax every day, she had no relief, and she had been hospitalized twice in the month preceding her first treatment due to the severity of the attacks. The chest pains terrified her. Basically, she was a wreck, overwhelmed, and unable to function in her day-to-day life anymore. Who could blame her?

Dawn had gone to the emergency room at least a dozen times. Medication did almost nothing to relieve her symptoms. She had difficulty working and taking care of her children and was afraid to drive. Before the panic attacks she said she felt fine emotionally. According to Dawn, they "came out of nowhere." Most panic attack sufferers say the exact same thing. Her sleep had been erratic for as long as she could remember. Dawn slept well maybe four nights out of seven. She woke up with her heart racing a few nights per week.

Dawn's nightmares would awaken her in a completely overwrought state. The more tired she was, the worse the panic attacks would be.

On top of suffering from panic attacks, Dawn had some other medical issues, including thinning hair and premature graying, irregular menses with heavy bleeding and severe cramps, rosacea on her nose and chin, weight problems, fatigue, low back pain, and headaches at the base of the skull at least once a month. Dawn told me she never felt completely well. She almost always had the sense that something was going wrong with her healthwise. If it wasn't her period, she was exhausted, or her back hurt. Dawn was never at 100 percent.

When it came to eating habits, Dawn unfortunately consumed the SAD diet. She ate lots of white bread, white rice, nothing organic, and rarely any fresh vegetables. She lived off cream cheese and bagels, cheese sticks, ice cream, french fries, diet soda, and macaroni and cheese from a box. Occasionally Dawn would eat a salad, usually from a fast food restaurant. Fast food or frozen dinners were the norm in her home. Coffee, in her mind, was as necessary as water, and a pot a day was the norm. She added several tablespoons of cream to each cup. As you learned earlier in chapter 7, coffee and caffeine can exacerbate any anxiety symptoms. Clearly her food choices needed a complete overhaul.

I focused on getting the panic attacks under control at first because they were so debilitating. Suspecting that food allergies might be a contributing factor to her panic attacks, I had her tested, and Dawn immediately stopped eating anything she was allergic to. She was allergic to all her favorite foods, so the elimination process was a challenge for Dawn, but she was willing to say good-bye to anything that was detrimental to her health.

She also gave up white foods except for potatoes. No more Wonder Bread or microwaved Uncle Ben's rice. Dawn started having fresh vegetables every day. Quinoa and root vegetables became her favorite things to eat. She actually looked forward to her morning green juice and lunchtime salad. The thought of McDonald's or nuking a frozen dinner was totally gross to her after a while, proof that your tastes can change.

Since she was highly motivated to feel better, Dawn was eager to incorporate kidney-boosting foods into her diet. "Anything to feel

The Calcium Conundrum

Another question I get asked a lot is "Don't you need milk for calcium?" The answer is a big no. Dairy foods actually do not have much calcium compared to plant foods (see below), and many people are allergic/lactose intolerant. This means they can't access the calcium in dairy anyway, and it can make them really sick. Dairy has also been linked to heart disease, prostate cancer, and Type II diabetes.

The dairy industry spent almost $200 million in advertising in 2011 in the United States alone. So that's pretty much why everyone believes you can only get enough calcium from eating dairy: marketing. The guys from *Mad Men* would be proud.

A staggering statistic that also disproves this myth: On average, Americans eat the most dairy, yet have the highest rates of osteoporosis. According to the Wisconsin Milk Marketing Board, we eat almost three hundred pounds of dairy per year per person.

Besides not providing high levels of calcium, eating a lot of dairy and animal protein makes your body acidic. To alkalize itself after consuming acidic foods, the body leeches calcium from your bones. Stress, inactivity, exposure to toxins, and eating acidic foods, such as processed foods, meat, sugar, and coffee, can lead to a whole host of illnesses, not just osteoporosis. Possible consequences of an acidic lifestyle are weight gain, low energy, hormonal imbalances, and depression. The main reason for this is that the body can't assimilate nutrients or heal itself when it's acidic.

Native Eskimos have the highest dietary calcium intake of any people in the world—above 2,000 milligrams per day from fish bones. Their diet is also the highest in protein in the world—up to 400 grams per day, primarily from fish. Yet native Eskimos have the highest rates of osteoporosis in the world.

On the other hand, the largely vegetarian African Bantu peoples consume an average of only 350 milligrams of calcium per day, yet do not have calcium deficiency, seldom break a bone, and rarely lose a tooth. There are two theories for this: One, we don't need as much calcium as the National Dairy Council tells us, and two, the Bantu eat easy-to-absorb sources of calcium and minimal acidic foods. Their diet mainly consists of calcium-rich foods such as millet, sweet potatoes, sorghum, and beans. I think the reason for the Bantus' bone health is a combination of the two. The amount we supposedly need assumes most Americans are contributing to the weakening of their bones through our incredibly unhealthy and sedentary lifestyles. Our bones and teeth are begging for more calcium.

Still don't believe me? Look at these numbers.

Calcium Sources

In milligrams per 100-gram serving

Butter	20
Whole milk	118

Chickpeas	150
Collard greens	203
Parsley	203
Soybeans	226
Almonds	234
Sesame seeds	1,160

In milligrams per 8 ounces (1 cup)

Soybean sprouts	50
Mung bean sprouts	35
Alfalfa sprouts	25
Nori	1,200
Kombu	2,100
Wakame	3,500
Tofu	350
Quinoa	80
Kale	72
Okra	81
Cornmeal	50
Oats	40
Carrot juice	57
Navy beans	140
Pinto beans	100
Lima beans	60
Black beans	60
Lentils	50
Hazelnuts	450
Walnuts	280
Sunflower seeds	260

Recommended Daily Allowance

0–6 months	200 milligrams
6–12 months	260 milligrams
1–3 years	700 milligrams
4–8 years	1,000 milligrams
9–18 years	1,300 milligrams
19–50 years	1,000 milligrams
Pregnant/lactating women	1,300 milligrams
51–70 years, male	1,000 milligrams
51–70 years, female	1,200 milligrams
70+ years	1,200 milligrams

So as you can see, the "milk does the body good" campaign just isn't true. Do yourself a favor. Go to your local farmers' market. Try some fresh, green veggies. Buy yourself a juicer and enjoy. Grab a handful of almonds. Eat some hummus. Your bones will thank you.

better" was her attitude. Here's just a sample of the foods I recommended Dawn incorporate into her eating routine.

Breakfast: smoothie with blackberries, unsweetened hemp milk, Vega One powder, chia seeds, and mango.

Lunch: vegan coleslaw with red and green cabbage and Vegenaise; half sandwich with sprouted Ezekiel bread, broccoli sprouts, and black bean hummus.

Snacks: miso soup with carrots, radish, sesame seeds, and tofu. (Dawn brought a thermos of it to work.)

Dinner: chili with black beans and a beet salad.

Dawn's progress was astonishing. There was an immediate reduction in the frequency of the panic attacks. The intensity diminished within a few weeks. Dawn never felt the need to go to the hospital again after coming to see me. Whenever she felt the hint of anxiety, she took her herbs and instantly felt relief. Last I heard from her, she hadn't had a panic attack in five years. She also lost fifteen pounds and was getting her periods regularly. She continued therapy to help deal with the issues that led to her attacks.

Recap of Dawn's Water-related symptoms: panic attacks, headaches, adrenal fatigue, premature graying.

There are plenty of delicious, healthy options for supporting your kidneys and reducing anxiety. Whether it's purple potatoes or quinoa, give something new a try every week! (But please consult your doctor before stopping any medications.) You'll feel the fear lift and an abatement in any kidney-related issues. Anxiety and panic attacks don't have to last a lifetime. Wendy and Dawn were able to experience some relief right away. I used them as examples because they were proactive in their healing process and both overcame so much. And so can you!

PART III

Western World

He who takes medicine and neglects to diet wastes the skill of his doctors.
—CHINESE PROVERB

CHAPTER 12

Western Nutrition for Mental Health

Every vitamin and mineral you ingest can impact your mood. Of course, getting enough of all your nutrients is very important to your physical health as well. Balanced hormones, optimal brain function, and the strength and purity of your blood are key factors to improving your state of mind. As you learned earlier, there are certain ingredients to stay away from to avoid energy crashes and moodiness. You also want to make sure you get ample amounts of what you really need to stay calm, cool, and collected. It's important to know what nutrients to pay attention to when feeling low. Many times, a vitamin deficiency or not enough healthy bacteria in the digestive tract can be major contributors to mental health issues.

Though I am a strong believer in TCM, I have seen many patients who have benefited from simple dietary changes based on Western science. A lack in nutrients can be the main, if not only, cause of many disagreeable moods. My patient Mary was one memorable example. She found herself following every extreme diet ever published for almost twenty years. She did the cabbage diet, the grapefruit diet, the master cleanse for two months instead of ten days, the no-carb diet, the no-fat diet, the HCG (human growth hormone) 500-calorie-a-day diet, and the Special K diet.

Mary took laxatives, fen-phen, amphetamines, and daily enemas and laxatives. She admitted to spending a ten-month period consuming only 1,000 calories a day and working out two hours daily. You name it, she probably tried it. Mary had done so many failed diets, she had thought about writing a book on her yo-yo weight-loss insanity. Her constantly changing attempts to lose weight were particularly sad because Mary wasn't all that heavy—just about twenty-five pounds overweight.

Every time she did one of these detrimental diets, she felt absolutely horrible, obsessed about food, and usually gained every pound back within a couple of months. Mary told me her mood swings were horrendous, intense fatigue was the norm, PMS made her a raving lunatic, and she was perpetually battling depression. She simply wasn't consuming enough nutrients. Her body and brain were starving. It's no wonder her emotional state was so grim.

Most fad diets are lacking in sound nutritional advice and aren't sustainable—mentally or physically. Depending on which diet Mary was on would determine what she was deficient in. She was always deprived of her B vitamins, calories, and fiber. The no-fat diets always meant she wasn't consuming enough healthy fat. The no-carb diet lead to an inadequate intake of fiber. Mary wasn't even allowed to have broccoli on that one. Her doctor at the time told her broccoli contributed to weight gain because it is high in carbohydrates!

Mary would drink a six-pack of diet soda a day for energy. She was so exhausted from malnourishment that it was her only way to function at work. She believed soda, especially diet, couldn't be that bad. A few doctors even suggested Mary drink it to increase energy and aid in her weight loss.

Once Mary had been on a balanced plant-based diet for a few months, along with acupuncture every two weeks and daily herbs, she became a new person. She was calmer, happier, and achieved her goal weight in just three months. Eight years later, Mary is still doing well.

I could easily write a book on how each vitamin and mineral is used in the body, how they support you emotionally, and how to find them. Every nutrient we consume, or should consume, plays an important part in mood. But I would like to focus on four essential elements in any diet: iron, B vitamins, vitamin D, and healthy fats.

IRON

Iron is a nutrient most associated with beef. Let's debunk that myth right now. A 100-calorie piece of sirloin steak has 0.8 milligram of iron, while 100 calories of spinach has 15.5 milligrams, and lentils 2.9 milligrams.

There are two forms of iron, heme and nonheme. Heme iron is easier to absorb and makes up 40 percent of the iron in meat, poultry, and fish. Nonheme iron is in all plant food sources and makes up 60 percent of the iron in meats and fish. Vegans and vegetarians don't have higher rates of iron deficiency than their meat-eating friends, because most fruits and vegetables have a significant amount of vitamin C, which aids in the absorption of iron. Iron-rich foods like kale, bok choy, and brussels sprouts all have an abundance of C. Even C-rich watermelon has iron in it.

Iron makes red blood cells and aids in the transportation of oxygen and cell growth. It does this by helping the blood move oxygen from the lungs to the tissue cells where it is needed. That's why fatigue and muscle weakness are two of the most obvious symptoms of anemia.

Are you getting enough iron? Your body will probably tell you when it needs you to load up on spinach and lentil soup. Symptoms of iron deficiency include insomnia, irritability, pale skin and nail beds, fatigue, dizziness, weakness, shortness of breath, sore tongue and mouth, light-headedness, brittle nails, decreased appetite (especially in children), and headaches. Other symptoms include heartburn, gas, vague abdominal pains, numbness and tingling in the extremities, heart palpitations, and sores at the corners of the mouth. Women need to pay attention to whether or not any of the above symptoms increase during or right after their periods. That's usually a sign of anemia.

In Chinese medicine, not having enough blood in the liver is the same as anemia. Most of the time I'm able to diagnose and treat anemia without a blood test. Blood deficiency of the liver leads to blood deficiency in the rest of the body. There are some emotional issues associated specifically with liver blood deficiency. They include panic attacks, insomnia, anxiety, mood swings, emotional sensitivity, and volatility. In TCM it is thought that the soul needs strong, nutrient-rich blood to protect it and to rest. So it makes sense that Western medicine agrees with some of the possible manifestations of iron-poor blood.

Wendy (from chapter 11) had been anemic since her teenage years due to her history of eating disorders. Even though she had been in recovery for bulimia and anorexia for a number of years, she was still anemic. Her digestive tract was so damaged that it had a difficult time taking in the nutrients she was eating. Once Wendy's digestion was working properly, her insomnia and anxiety decreased right away.

What causes the malabsorption of iron? Along with deficient intake of vitamin C, there are a few other causes. In men and post-menopausal women, anemia is usually due to blood loss associated with ulcers; eating disorders; the overuse of aspirin or nonsteroidal anti-inflammatory medications (NSAIDS); consuming coffee, tea, calcium-rich foods, or vitamins too close to consuming iron-rich foods or supplements; or colon cancer.

Iron is mostly absorbed from the duodenum (part of the intestines) and upper small intestine. So if you have any digestive issues such as gas, constipation, bloating, celiac disease, Crohn's disease, or food sensitivities, you could be at risk for anemia.

Phytate, which is found in some whole grains and legumes, can limit iron absorption. Soy, which is a good vegetarian source of iron, contains phytate and certain proteins that unfortunately interfere with iron absorption. Other foods that obstruct iron absorption include coffee, tea (including some herbal), cocoa, calcium, and some spices. Keep in mind that only 15 percent of the iron we consume is absorbed. To give you an example, if you eat 15 milligrams of iron per day, your body is only absorbing about 2.25 milligrams.

Some iron loss occurs naturally. The total daily iron loss of an adult is about 1 milligram, and about 2 milligrams in women during menstruation. Children, men, and women have different nutritional needs based on their ages. See the chart below for guidelines.

Daily Iron Requirements

Children

7 months–1 year	11 milligrams
1 year–4 years	7 milligrams
4 years–8 years	10 milligrams
9 years–13 years	8 milligrams

Women

14–50 years	10–15 milligrams
51+ years	8 milligrams
Pregnant	30 milligrams
Lactating	10 milligrams

Men

14+ years	10 milligrams

Sources of Iron

Food (1 cup)	Iron (in mg)	Food (1 cup)	Iron (in mg)
Black beans	7.9	Tofu	4.6
Garbanzos	6.9	Lima beans	4.5
Pinto beans	6.1	Lentils	6.6
Navy beans	5.1	Split peas	3.4
Soybeans	8.8	Fresh peas	2.9
Kidney beans	5.2	Tempeh	2.2
Vegetables (1 cup cooked)			
Spinach	6.4	Kale	1.8
Beet greens	2.8	Acorn squash	1.7
Swiss chard	4.0	Brussels sprouts	1.7
Tomato juice	2.2	Potato with skin	1.4
Butternut squash	2.1	Beets	1.0
Fruit			
Prune juice, 1 cup	10.5	Dates, 10	2.4
Dried peach halves, 5	3.9	Prunes, 1 cup	1.8
Raisins, ½ cup	2.6	Strawberries, 1 cup	1.5
Grains (¼ cup dry)			
Rice bran	10.8	Wheat bran/germ	1.9
Quinoa	4.6	Cream of wheat	8.1
Millet	3.9	Oat- or cornmeal	0.7
Seeds (¼ cup)			
Pumpkin seeds	4.0	Sunflower seeds	2.4
Miscellaneous			
Blackstrap molasses, 1 tablespoon	3.2	Brewer's yeast, 1 tablespoon	1.4
Tahini, 2 tablespoons	2.7	Cashews, ¼ cup	2.0

INTRO TO YOUR B VITAMINS

B vitamins, once thought to be just one vitamin, are actually eight very distinct nutrients that promote your mental health. B vitamins, especially B_{12}, are great for the nervous system and supporting the adrenal glands. What does this mean? When you are balanced in your B vitamins and faced with a tough time or high stress at work or home, you'll feel calmer, more even-keeled. Taking them together, in a B complex, will give you optimal results. All B vitamins are water soluble. This means you pee out what you don't need every day, and your body doesn't hold on to any reserves. So getting enough of your Bs every day is key.

Vitamin B_1, or thiamine, is vital to balanced mental health and nourishing your nervous system. It improves memory, stabilizes your mood, and converts glucose into energy. Sources include sunflower seeds, flaxseeds, brussels sprouts, navy beans, black beans, pinto beans, lentils, peas, sesame seeds, lima beans, and spinach.

B_2 is also known as riboflavin. It aids in the metabolism of carbohydrates and fats, maintains the levels of all the other B vitamins, and protects cells from oxidation. Riboflavin assists in the energy production of cells. Sources include spinach, soybeans, mushrooms, almonds, collard greens, and green peas.

A deficiency of Vitamin B_3, or niacin, can lead to depression, irritability, and other mood disorders. It helps optimize the functions of digestion and the nervous system. By helping the release of energy from carbohydrates, niacin can help control blood-sugar levels. Sources include spelt, peanuts, mushrooms, broccoli, brown rice, and tomatoes.

B_5, also known as pantothenic acid, enhances the production of healthy fats in the body and improves the immune system. It also helps metabolize fat and carbohydrates to be used as energy. Sources include cauliflower, broccoli, grapefruit, mushrooms, avocado, corn, sweet potato, bell peppers, and asparagus.

Vitamin B_6 plays a role in the biosynthesis of important neurotransmitters: serotonin, epinephrine, norepinephrine, dopamine, and gamma-aminobutyric acid. They are imperative to brain function. For example, low levels of serotonin can cause insomnia and depression. Dopamine is released when we feel happy or experience pleasure, and it is responsible for regulating appetite, sleep, memory, temperature, mood, muscle contraction, and function of the cardio-vascular system and endocrine system. B_6 is necessary for the brain to produce adequate amounts of dopamine and other neurotransmitters. Low blood levels of B_6 have been linked to symptoms of depression. B_6 also improves immunity. Sources include peanuts, soybeans, walnuts, bananas, watermelon, bell peppers, summer squash, sunflower seeds, spinach, avocado, and turnip greens.

Biotin, or vitamin B_7, is key in metabolizing fat and carbohydrates. It also helps with enhancing mood. Biotin is crucial in processing glucose. This also means that Type II diabetics would benefit from taking biotin to aid in regulating blood sugar levels. Sources include nutritional yeast, walnuts, peanuts, oatmeal, mushrooms, soy, broccoli, cauliflower, and spinach.

Vitamin B_9, which is also called folic acid, increases energy. It also protects the heart and brain, helps in the production of red blood cells, prevents cell damage that may lead to certain cancers, and reduces depression and increases efficacy of some antidepressants. Sources include lentils, pinto beans, garbanzo beans, spinach, collard and turnip greens, kidney and navy beans, beets, parsley, broccoli, asparagus, romaine lettuce, and lima beans.

B_{12}, along with helping brain function, has an important role in the formation of blood. It is involved in the metabolism of every cell of the body, especially affecting DNA synthesis and regulation, but also fatty acid synthesis and energy production. B_{12} is critical in the production of melatonin and serotonin.

If you're leaning toward going vegan or vegetarian, or are already there, you'll need to take a B_{12} supplement. It should be made with methylcobalamin, which is more readily used by your body. I like to cook with nutritional yeast, which is fortified with B vitamins, including B_{12}. Nutritional yeast has a nutty flavor and is delicious in most savory recipes.

B vitamins in general help support and increase the metabolic rate, maintain healthy skin and muscle tone, enhance immune and nervous system function, and promote cell growth and division, including that of the red blood cells that help prevent anemia.

A deficiency in B vitamins may have many causes, including alcoholism, autoimmune disorders such as lupus or Graves' disease, a lack of intrinsic factor that aids in absorption of B_{12} (i.e., long-term use of acid-reducing drugs or certain medications, kidney problems, or diseases of the small intestine such as Crohn's disease, celiac disease, bacterial overgrowth, or a parasite.

VITAMIN D: D IS FOR DEPRESSION

What is all this hype about vitamin D deficiency? It seems to be the new health trend. Most doctors didn't test for it or even ask about D until a couple of years ago. It turns out that insufficient vitamin D is a bit of an epidemic: Approximately 40 percent of Americans are vitamin D deficient.

So why is there such a problem? First, if you live north of Los Angeles on the West Coast or Florida on the East Coast, and north of those locations in the middle of the country, you can't get enough D from the sun in winter. If you work indoors, always wear sunblock, avoid going out in the sun, are obese, have kidney disease, or are over sixty, you are at high risk. (Sunscreens, while helpful for other things, block your ability to get D from the sun by up to 95 percent.)

Vitamin D is responsible for strengthening the immune system, bone and heart health, reducing cancer risk, muscle flexibility, calcium absorption, and mood elevation. Recent studies conclude that seasonal affective disorder (another SAD) may be related to D's impact on serotonin in the brain. Vitamin D also plays a part in the release in dopamine, another neurotransmitter related to our emotional state.

There are plenty of signs to signal that you might be vitamin D deficient. Some health consequences of not getting enough D include osteoporosis, arthritis, poor memory, easily fractured or broken bones, weak or sore muscles, autoimmune disease, prostate and breast cancer, frequent colds, depression, even the slightest pressure on your sternum is tender to the touch, impaired insulin production, and possibly even schizophrenia.

There are a few sources of vitamin D, but the best is the way nature intended, in the form of sunlight without sunblock for five to thirty minutes per day on the arms and legs; otherwise take a vegan D_3 supplement of 2,000 international units (IU) daily. Mushrooms, especially shiitake, and fortified organic soy milk also are good sources. Have you doctors check your vitamin D levels, especially if you're experiencing any symptoms mentioned above. Keep in mind that it can take months to replenish your vitamin D. Get outside and enjoy a little sun. It does the body good.

HEALTHY FATS MAKE YOU SMARTER

You need to eat some fat. Period. You can't live a truly healthy, well-balanced life without consuming at least some fat. Our organs can't optimally function without it. Did you know your brain is about 60 percent fat, and that your hormones are made from fat? Sixty percent of your heart's energy comes from burning fats. Your lungs need fat to work and to keep them from collapsing. Fats help you absorb certain vital nutrients, including fat-soluble vitamins A, D, E, and K.

I know there's plenty of confusing information out there about what's healthy to eat and what isn't. One myth is that all fat is bad all the time. Low-fat and nonfat products became all the rage in the 1990s and still exist today, but not all fats are created equal.

Monounsaturated fats are the healthy kind. The best-known example is olive oil, but don't cook with it. High temperatures change the chemical makeup of olive oil, which can make it carcinogenic (cancer causing). Eat olives instead. For cooking, I recommend sautéing in just a little vegetable broth. Some research shows that refined oils aren't a good idea to use at all. I definitely agree to limit the use of them.

There are plenty of tasty sources for healthy fat. These sources include walnuts, flaxseeds, hemp seeds, pumpkin seeds, and avocado. I recommend adding flax-, chia, or hemp seeds, plus some almond butter, to your morning smoothie. A surprising source of healthy fat is seaweed and sea vegetables. Seaweed is an excellent way to get your essential fatty acids. Why do you think fish are considered such a good source of healthy fat? It's from what they eat.

If you don't get enough healthy fat, you may experience depression, poor sleep/fatigue, impaired memory, difficulty concentrating, and a lack of mental clarity when you first get up in the morning. Though this is a chapter on nutrition and mental health, it's worth mentioning the physical symptoms as well, which include infertility, weight gain, brittle fingernails, allergies, arthritis, and dry hair and skin.

My diet-crazed patient Mary attempted eating fat-free for two years when she was twenty-five years old. Guess how she felt during those two years? She had irregular periods, could barely study for law school, her previously gorgeous long nails broke off easily, and she had a difficult time doing her normal routine at the gym. Other factors might have contributed to her symptoms, but eliminating all fat from her diet was a major cause.

TAKING VITAMINS: DO I OR DON'T I?

Even if you have the healthiest, cleanest vitamin-rich diet, you might not be getting all you need. Since our soils are so depleted, most produce doesn't provide the nutrients we would expect. The end result is that eating only whole foods isn't a guarantee that you're actually consuming enough nourishment.

A recent study in England found that the calcium content of modern vegetables is about one-fifth lower than what was measured in the 1960s, and average copper content declined almost 80 percent. Oranges have been shown to have only one-eighth the amount of vitamin A as two generations ago. One US study spanning 1963–1999 proved that, per 100 grams, tomatoes lost 8 milligrams of calcium, 3 milligrams of magnesium, and 22 milligrams of vitamin K. Other vegetables' numbers dropped dramatically too: iron levels 37 percent, vitamin A levels 21 percent, and vitamin C levels 30 percent.

Unless you're a locavore (someone who eats only locally grown foods), you're probably eating at least a portion of each meal from across the globe. Produce loses its nutrient content as soon as it's been picked—another reason to buy seasonally.

There's also a proliferation of causes that lead to a lack of absorption of nutrients. High stress, certain medications, food allergies, drinks (like coffee, energy drinks, and soda), irregular eating schedules, antacids, and antibiotics found in nonorganic animal products have wreaked havoc on our digestion. Our stomachs, spleens, and intestines are unable to function to their full capacity. They're in charge of absorbing all the nutrients we're taking in. The end result is malnutrition.

If you eat more of a SAD diet (hopefully not after reading this book), you'll definitely need some added nutritional support. Most, if not all, processed foods are just empty calories, meaning there's a ton of calories and nothing else. You might be eating 3,000 calories a day, but your body is starving. You crave more food, even though you're full. Once again, the end result is malnourishment.

With our lives the way they are today, most people probably have some days, weeks, or even months and years when they could be eating better. Of course, my preference is to eat only whole foods for nourishment, but not everyone is going to eat that way or have access to fresh produce. I encourage you to always do your best.

So sometimes you might need some additional support. If you're experiencing a health issue—thyroid disorder, frequent colds, allergies, chronic fatigue, depression, migraines, female issues—the right vitamins and herbal supplements can help you get back on track, or even help you feel better than you ever have before. Most of my patients and people I know are used to feeling a little bit under the weather, stressed, or exhausted all the time. Usually a natural boost is all that is required to experience major improvement.

I'm frequently asked if I think a certain brand of vitamins is any good. I definitely have my favorites, but there are so many brands on the market now, it would be impossible to research all of them. When I first started studying nutrition in high school, there were only a couple of brands sold at the few health food stores that existed. Now a few rows are dedicated to supplements, even at pharmacies. Unfortunately, buying most brands is like throwing your money away, and many can even make you sick.

Some companies are making some incredible claims. I'm skeptical of any that tout miracle cures: "Take our product for two weeks, and you'll be in perfect health." "You can eat and drink whatever you want. Just take these pills to lose weight and feel great." Usually when something sounds too good to be true, it *is* too good be true.

Most people just assume that taking any vitamin is a good thing. Unfortunately, this isn't always the case. Many companies are producing vitamins that can't be absorbed well, if at all. They can also come from toxic or inorganic (nonliving) sources. Some calcium supplements are just ground-up seashells. The thought is that seashells contain calcium, so they're a good source of calcium for humans. No, sorry. It doesn't work that way. What the human body can use and take in from nature is an exact science. Many vitamins even contain iron filings. Iron filings. Can anyone really think this is a good or even safe source for iron? Don't get me wrong, there are some great products out there, too. They're just few and far between.

Every nutrient you ingest raises or lowers up to nine other nutrients in your body. For example, taking large doses of vitamin C lowers your level of copper, so if you are already deficient in copper and take high doses of vitamin C, you can actually compromise your immune system. As you will read in the last chapter, vitamin C increases the absorption of iron. So make sure you're getting enough copper and eat an orange or drink some lemon water with your iron supplement.

What should you look for in a vitamin supplement? Safe sources. I prefer vitamins and supplements from plant-based whole foods. Ideally, they should be organic as well. Not all plants are available as organic just yet. The more consumers demand them, the sooner companies will want to sell them, and the sooner farmers will grow them. The more a plant is chemically processed, the less available the nutrients will be. Sometimes my patients are surprised when I recommend a special formula that requires nine pills per day. This is because the herbs I use aren't altered to be condensed into one tiny pill. We're used to this with medications, but this process isn't beneficial when it comes to herbs.

What should you avoid? If you're taking a supplement that has been chemically processed and isolated, most likely your body won't be able to metabolize it. It might even make you sick. A vitamin might claim that it has 100 percent or more of what you need in a day, but if you don't absorb much or any of it, you're wasting your money. If a vitamin has extra-high doses, say 200 percent of vitamin A, it can actually become poisonous to your system. Our bodies can't flush out excess amounts of oil-soluble vitamins A, D, E, and K, so an overabundant amount of certain nutrients will build up in your body and become toxic. Symptoms of vitamin A toxicity include headaches, nausea, dizziness, itchy skin, osteoporosis, joint pain, visual disturbances, and even swelling of the brain. I know the Western mentality is "more equals better," but when taking supplements, this is rarely the case.

You should also watch out for other ingredients. Are there any animal products in the supplement? Safety regulations aren't strong enough at this point. Many fish oils come from fish that are loaded with mercury. Bovine (cow) and other animal sources aren't tested for mad cow disease, other illnesses, or bacteria like salmonella and *E. coli*. So if you are taking any supplements from animal sources, please do your research on how the company does its quality testing.

Also watch out for dangerous fillers. If at all possible steer clear of vitamins or supplements with any of the words in the list below on the label; these are some of the most commonly used binders and fillers in drugs, vitamins, minerals, and supplements, but unfortunately they're not always listed. They can all be detrimental to your health.

Propylene glycol	Talc
Lactose	Sucrose
Starch	Povidone
Pregelatinized starch	Cellulose
Hydroxypropyl	Methycellulose
Silicon dioxide	Calcium phosphate
Calcium stearate	Hydroxypropyl cellulose
Stearic acid	Ethylcellulose
Sodium starch	Glycolate
BHT	Polysorbate 80
Microcrystalline cellulose	Tartrazine
Red dye 33 and 40	Peanut oil
Hydrogenated cottonseed oil	Fractionated coconut oil
Fractionated cornstarch	Sodium benzoate
Partially hydrogenated soybean oil	Sodium lauryl sulfate
Sodium laureth sulfate	

Can you believe these ingredients are in products that are supposed to promote health? Here is some more detail about a few of these ingredients, just so you can begin to get an idea of how bad they really are.

Today, pretty much anyone who follows nutrition knows that **hydrogenated oils** are harmful, and that long-term consumption will lead to cardiovascular disease and heart attacks. They can even encourage strokes. We know that they cause harm, sometimes irreparable, to the nervous system. Hydrogenated oils interfere with the absorption of the essential fatty acids.

Propylene glycol is commonly used as antifreeze and is an ingredient in windshield washer fluid, brake fluid, and hydraulic fluid. It is also found in cosmetics, deodorants, shampoos, and lotions. It causes liver and kidney damage. Do you really want this in your vitamin?

Sodium lauryl sulfate (SLS) and **sodium laureth sulfate (SLES)** are used for their cleaning and foaming abilities. These are found in garage floor cleaners, car wash soap, engine degreasers, and personal care products like shampoo. SLS and SLES can form carcinogenic nitrates and dioxins, all of which may enter the circulation with shampooing or ingesting.

SLS can be stored in the liver, heart, eyes, kidneys, and muscles for several years after use and has been known to cause skin rashes, dandruff, allergic reactions, hair loss, and eye irritations. Do you really want to put something supposedly natural in your body if only a chemist knows what it is?

These tips should take you further on your path to wellness. I've only given a few examples of mood-boosting nutrients in this chapter. To guarantee good health and a carefree state of mind, make sure to eat a rainbow of food every day. Now you also have more tools when you need some additional guidance in the vitamin and supplement aisle. If you're unsure what to look for, ask for help from the person who is in charge of the supplement section at your market. Bring the above list with you. Vitamins and herbal supplements should be an addition to your already health-promoting eating plan. They can add to the already strong foundation of a balanced diet.

The greatest wealth is health.

—Virgil

CHAPTER 13

Why Organic?

After you learn how to choose the right foods, the next step is going organic. Until the twentieth century, there was no need to talk about "organic" food. All food was organic, and pesticide residue and artificial preservatives were unknown. People didn't have to think about what might be in the bread they bought from the town baker, or if their greens might be doing more harm than good. Food was food.

Some people in my life may say I am a bit anal about what I eat. They might be right. I still get eye rolls from loved ones for refusing gum with fake sugar or a drink mixed with Coke. But I have very good reasons for wanting my food and supplements to be as clean as possible. I realize getting all of your food—or even some of it—organic might not be an option, either because of money constraints or because it's just not available where you live. So do your best!

Why go organic? Nonorganic means genetically modified, antibiotics, growth hormones, and/or pesticides and herbicides, none of which are safe for consumption. The term *genetically modified organism* (GMO) means that foreign DNA has been forced into a plant or seed. Genetic engineering even transfers genes across natural species barriers. One company tried to get the US Food and Drug

Administration's approval to sell a tomato that included genes from a winter flounder. Yes, fish DNA forced into a tomato. But most, if not all, GMOs contain microorganisms such as bacteria and yeast, as well as insects, plants, fish, and mammals.

The most common genetically modified foods are corn, soy, cottonseed, alfalfa (fed to dairy cows), canola, and sugar beets. Studies prove that GMOs increase breast cancer risk, tumor growth and instances of food allergies, especially to soy and gluten. I had a big "aha" moment about GMOs and allergies while doing my residency. A French patient of mine commented that whenever she went to visit family in France, eating baguettes and croissants didn't upset her stomach. But in the States, she felt gassy and sluggish every time she ate a sandwich. This is most likely because France has some of the strictest laws about limiting and banning GMO crops.

To add to the frustration about food safety, there are chemical pesticides and herbicides. More than seventeen thousand pesticide products are currently on the market in the US. The average American consumes three pounds of pesticides per year. This is particularly scary when you consider that your brain weighs about three pounds. If you limit or completely eliminate nonorganic food from your grocery basket, your exposure to chemicals will be limited as well.

Concern about pesticides has driven many people to go organic. Pesticides can have quite a few negative consequences on your health. I'm always surprised that most pesticides are even legal. Many of the illnesses we consider unavoidable and part of the norm can be traced back to being subjected to pesticides. The human health impacts linked to pesticide exposure range from birth defects and childhood brain cancer in the very young to Parkinson's disease in the elderly. In between are a variety of other cancers, developmental and neurological disorders, reproductive and hormonal system disruptions, and more. Pesticides are suspected as a possible contributing factor to autism, ADD/ADHD, hormonal imbalances, gestational diabetes, infertility, thyroid disorders, obesity, and delayed puberty in boys.

When it comes to produce, some nonorganic options are safer than others because certain fruits and vegetables absorb more pesticides. So just washing them well isn't really enough to get rid of any residue. Please use this list when doing your shopping.

THE TWELVE MOST POLLUTED TYPES OF PRODUCE (AKA THE DIRTY DOZEN)

- Peaches
- Apples
- Sweet bell peppers
- Celery
- Nectarines
- Strawberries
- Cherries
- Pears
- Grapes
- Spinach
- Lettuce
- Potatoes

THE TWELVE LEAST POLLUTED TYPES OF PRODUCE

- Onions
- Avocado
- Sweet corn
- Pineapple
- Mangos
- Asparagus
- Sweet peas
- Kiwi fruit
- Bananas
- Cabbage
- Broccoli
- Papaya

Just as important for better health is avoiding plastic. You're probably saying to yourself, "Avoid using plastic? Why? I recycle, and it's so convenient! And how? It's *everywhere!*" If you went through every room and every cabinet, closet, and drawer, you would find plastic. It's in our clothes. It's the packaging for almost everything we buy. It's in our cars. Our toothbrushes and brushes are made of plastic. We can't get away from it.

Besides polluting our oceans and killing sea creatures and birds, plastic has been suspected as a cause of brain damage, increased fat formation and obesity risk, hyperactivity, increased aggressiveness, learning impairment, autoimmune disorders, early puberty, thyroid disorders, prostate enlargement, low sperm count, and various cancers. If you're experiencing any of the above symptoms, it may from your exposure and use of plastic.

I know these side effects might seem scary and overwhelming. I also know that it's almost impossible to avoid using all plastics. But doing regular detoxes, sweating, getting plenty of clean water, eating nutritious foods, and taking the proper supplements can help prevent, eliminate, and reduce the chance of having any of the above health issues.

To minimize your exposure to plastics, store your food in glass containers, use cooking oils in glass bottles, drink filtered water in a metal container, do not microwave foods that are in plastic containers or covered by plastic (ideally do not microwave at all), and make sure to take reusable bags each time you go to the grocery store. And please recycle!

I don't want to scare you—but at the same time I do. Minimizing exposure to pesticides, plastics, and GMOs is something we can all do. Ask your grocery store to carry more organic options. Any time you eat out, let the restaurant staff know you're interested in organic fare. Bring your own utensils to picnics and potlucks and refuse to drink out of a plastic straw at restaurants. Tell your elected representatives you demand safe food choices. Your voice will be heard. And this will benefit all of us.

A sad soul can kill you quicker than a germ.

—JOHN STEINBECK

CHAPTER 14

Let the Healing Begin

With all this knowledge, you are now on the road to recovery. When healing and releasing suppressed illnesses, emotions, and experiences, most people go through what is called a "healing crisis" or "healing reaction." Symptoms of this can be mild, such as a headache that lasts a day. Or more severe health concerns may arise, like vomiting or symptoms of bronchitis. The theory is that old injuries, illnesses, or discomforts, be they physical, emotional, or mental, must all be cleared out physically for the patient to be well. Every experience we have is stored in each of our cells. So when we really let go, our cells will flush out emotional and/or physical toxins.

For example, chronic strep throat in childhood treated with antibiotics several times can manifest as a sore throat when you are making the transition to a healthier you. It should pass within a couple of days.

Or if you are processing some painful experiences that contributed to your anxiety or depression, you may feel these emotions more intensely. Old memories might show up in your dreams. Even events that you don't remember at all can rise to the surface, creating intense, vivid dreams or flashbacks. I promise you this is a really good sign.

My patient Jerry (from chapter 10), who lost his daughter, had a few remarkable experiences while processing his grief. During his first acupuncture treatment, he saw his daughter in the room with him. The room was dark, but he could still see her, smiling and giggling. He told me he felt she was saying it was OK to move on. Several of my patients have seen loved ones who have passed during their treatments.

Jerry also started having daily migraines after three weeks of treatment and dietary changes. The headaches lasted six days. After the third day, he remembered that he had migraines every day for eight months after his daughter's death. He was loaded up on prescription painkillers the entire time, so he had never really had a chance to feel them before. After six days of suffering, he felt relief from his heartache as well as his headaches.

Susan (chapter 8), who lost her husband, had a similar experience after a few weeks of acupuncture. She developed fifteen canker sores on the inside of her mouth that lasted twenty-four hours. She said she had painful canker sores for weeks after her husband died.

Any of the following problems may occur during a healing crisis.

1. You may be more sensitive emotionally, easily angered, impatient, anxious, depressed, or cry for "no reason." For women, this may feel like intense PMS.
2. You may have various kinds of discharges, including pimples, boils, herpes outbreak, black feces, canker sores, body odors, rashes, and nasal and vaginal secretions. This sounds gross, but remember, it's temporary.
3. An old illness may return. Either the body didn't fully recover or the infection was suppressed with certain medications. This could be the strep throat I mentioned earlier, or a bladder infection, stomach bug, or chest cold.
4. You may experience a temporary change in menstruation. This shouldn't last more than a month or two.
5. Pain from old injuries you thought were healed might return to finally say good-bye in the form of headaches or muscle tension.
6. Digestive disturbances such as gas, bloating, constipation, and diarrhea may pay a visit.

7. You may feel especially weak or fatigued. Letting go of painful memories can be exhausting. If you're feeling tired, then you should rest.
8. Lower libido is a common occurrence for people who experienced sexual trauma or acted out sexually in their past.
9. You're literally shedding dead weight, so weight loss may occur. If you actually need to lose weight, it will most likely stay off. If you're already thin, the weight should come back.
10. You may experience a change in sleep patterns. Dreams that bring up old memories and emotions will happen for most. You might have some insomnia issues or need more sleep while you're mending.

One simple and affordable way to aid the healing and detox process is Epsom salts. There's nothing better than a steamy, relaxing soak in winter after a long, stressful day when your muscles are tense from a long day at work. So take twenty minutes to just soak in a hot bath with a few cups of Epsom salts to feel better. The therapeutic effects of Epsom salts include easing stress by replenishing magnesium (magnesium helps produce serotonin, a mood-elevating chemical), flushing out toxins and heavy metals, relieving cold symptoms, relaxing muscles and reducing inflammation, relieving asthma symptoms, preventing hardening of the arteries, and making insulin more effective by balancing magnesium and sulfate levels.

Epsom salts can also be taken internally with some water for constipation. I have to warn you about the taste, but if you're prone to constipation, it can really help. If you're looking to do a gallbladder cleanse, here's one recipe; try to do it when you can be near a bathroom the next day. Drink this concoction at night. It will definitely get things moving.

½ cup extra virgin olive oil
4 ounces fresh lime, lemon, or grapefruit juice
4 tablespoons Epsom salts

Go ahead and splurge on a three-dollar container of Epsom salts. You deserve it, and your body will thank you.

Be aware of how you're feeling and what you dream about while going through the healing process. This might help give you some insight on where your anger or fear is coming from. This awareness can only advance the process of a new you. So if you experience any of the above symptoms while making dietary changes, it's totally normal. If it gets to be overwhelming, slow down a bit. Make the changes more gradual. Be gentle with yourself. This should reduce your response.

If a healing crisis does occur, do your best to ride it out, especially if you end up with physical symptoms. Taking medications may push what's being released back down. Once you get to the other side, you'll know it was definitely worth a day or two of discomfort.

PART IV

Putting It All Together

Be not afraid of growing slowly, be afraid only of standing still.

—CHINESE PROVERB

CHAPTER 15

Taking Action

Congratulations! You're well on your way to a more tranquil, more serene you. Aren't you excited? Now that you have all these new tools and insights, the journey to feeling healthier has begun. The first step was reading this book. Now the rest is up to you.

Here are my top tips for using what you have learned and how to keep moving forward:

- Take action now. Don't wait until tomorrow, or when you have a week off from work. Start today! Want to really push yourself? Write down goals you'd like to achieve every day, every week, and every month for a year. Plan to reach those targets.

- Set practical goals and write them down. Cut back to one cup of coffee a day by the end of the month. Try to lose thirty pounds by next summer. Make a list of all the fresh, healthy produce you are going to buy at the farmers' market this weekend.

- Each morning when you wake up, remind yourself to keep your commitments. Keep an open mind and stay positive. Start your day with the attitude that you will succeed in not eating three doughnuts at the office today or that you will make the time to journal.

- Find some friends or family members to go on this journey with you, but make sure they are as committed as you are to improving their lives. If they're not truly ready, they might start to slack off. Their lack of dedication will make it all too tempting for you to go back to your old habits as well.

- Share your goals with your loved ones, knowing that most of them will be supportive. Embrace those who cheer you on, but be wary of anyone who resists your change or thinks you are just going through a phase. Some resistance from friends and family is inevitable, but you need to forge on, knowing you are changing for the better. It's not that the cynics don't love you; they're just used to the old you. If encouragement from family or friends isn't an option, find it elsewhere, through a life coach, a twelve-step program, a support group, a therapist, or a new friend.

- Keep in mind that there can be some bumps in the road. When you feel like giving up, don't. Making lifestyle changes and letting go of old behaviors can be challenging. But the payoff is huge.

- Be patient. Really letting go of old emotional garbage takes some time and effort. If you feel like you're taking two steps forward and one step back for a while, keep going. Or if your progress isn't happening fast enough for you, remind yourself that you're on the right path and keep at it. If your life has been out of balance for several years, changes won't happen overnight.

- Write a list of accomplishments and things for which you are grateful. What you write doesn't have to be earth-shattering: *Found an easy parking space just now. Resisted stopping for a cheeseburger. I love my job. My neighbor offered to help take care of my animals while I go out of town this weekend. I slept an extra half hour last night.* If you're feeling low or stuck, take out this list. It's important to remember how far you've come.

- If you give in to cravings and indulge in a weekend of depravity, that's OK. You've let off steam. Just get back on track and don't give up. It will only make you feel worse if you beat yourself up. None of us are perfect. The longer you're eating right, the less appealing sugar and processed foods will become.

- Make a copy of the food lists in this book that apply to you and keep them with you. This way you'll know what to order when you're out to eat or for last-minute grocery shopping on the way home from work.

- If you know a couple of people who've read this book, organize potlucks. You can share your recipes and why you used the ingredients you did. This might sound silly, but it's actually a lot of fun.

- Pick a half hour to an hour once a month to research new recipes that include your mood-supporting foods. Put this task in your calendar and follow through—no excuses. Your cooking repertoire will expand quickly.

- Make menus for the week or month. Make a plan that you know you'll stick to.

- Be prepared for healthy snacking at home and at work. If you always have mood-supporting snacks on hand, then there's no justification to cheat. Nuts, seeds, trail mix ingredients, and nut butters are available year-round. Also stock up on seasonal fruit, and prep carrot, celery, and bell pepper sticks at the beginning of the week. Have hummus and other dips in your office. With lots of healthy alternatives close at hand, you won't be tempted (or at least not as much) to dig into the box of doughnuts in the break room or sample the candy in your kitchen cabinet.

- Healthy meals don't happen magically; they take planning. Make a large pot of soup, stew, or a casserole on Sunday night to last most of the workweek. Also cook up a batch of quinoa or rice and prewash your kale and other greens so you can just grab them out of the fridge and dig in. You'll have ready-to-go meals, so when you're too hungry, busy, or tired to think about washing and chopping, all you'll have to do is reheat on your stovetop or in the oven.

- Start a journal to keep track of your progress. It will help you observe how you're feeling on a particular day and what foods made you feel better or worse. Note your mood when you wake up, after meals or snacks, and throughout the day. If you remember your dreams, keep track of any recurring themes. See if there's any connection between the dreams and what you ate that day.

- Find a licensed acupuncturist in your area. It's best to do this by referral. Ask friends, neighbors, and coworkers whom they recommend. If the first person you go to doesn't feel like a good fit, try someone new. Make sure they have experience treating mental health. Many acupuncturists specialize, just like MDs, and some might only treat pain, digestion, or gynecological issues. The right fit is important for getting the best results, especially when it comes to emotional release treatments.

- Alternate weeks, adding a healthy item to your diet one week and taking an unhealthy one out the next. You know your limits. Push yourself to improve, but not to the point of wanting to give up. If I can go from being addicted to SpaghettiOs, bacon, cheese, and ice cream to craving kale salad and beet juice, so can you.

- Let yourself have a treat once every week or two for all the hard work and the progress you're making. By treat, I mean get a massage or a mani/pedi, take a hike in the middle of the week, go to your favorite museum, or take a day trip. You definitely deserve it.

- Get to know the vendors at your farmers' market. They'll start to know what you like and make suggestions, and they can help you pick out the best they have to offer.

- Make sure your kitchen is set up to help you reach your goals. Get rid of all edibles in your cupboards that aren't part of your eating plan or beneficial to your progress. Restock your kitchen with items that will contribute to your health and healing process.

- Invest in a quality juicer and/or blender. If finances are tight, you can usually find refurbished ones online. Just think of all the money you'll save by not buying Starbucks every day. Commit to juicing every morning.

- Buy your legumes, nuts, and seeds in bulk. Make sure you have enough airtight glass containers. You can even use old pickle and peanut butter jars for storage.

While adjusting to this new way of living and eating, make sure to emphasize abundance over deprivation. Health-promoting food is delicious, and it can be rich, flavorful, creamy, and decadent. Just think how lucky you are to have this opportunity to feel better. You get to start over. If you feel you are depriving yourself, you will find it much harder to change your diet and lifestyle.

Now that you have all these great new tools and insights into your health, it's time to make changes. I can't stress this enough. Take advantage of this opportunity and make the time to heal and look inward. You may dredge up some pretty painful feelings and memories. Be gentle with yourself. As you start to feel better, you'll be invigorated and energized.

I hope my patients' stories have inspired you as much as they've inspired me.

Live natural. Live well.

Let food be thy medicine, and let thy medicine be food.
—HIPPOCRATES

The food you eat can be either the safest and most powerful form of medicine or the slowest form of poison.
—ANN WIGMORE

CHAPTER 16

Food, Glorious Food

Almost all whole foods have healing properties. I've picked some of the most common whole food choices and given you a list of some of their physical and mental benefits. It's really that simple. Eating unprocessed food will boost your mood, increase your energy levels, and prevent illness. All plant-based whole foods have restorative properties. You can't go wrong buying groceries exclusively from the produce department. For this chapter I've picked some of my favorites that are packed with nutrients, and given you a list of their physical and mental health benefits.

If a lot of these are really new to you, feel free to get creative. The more you experiment cooking with whole foods, the more you'll know what combinations you like best. Your palate will gradually change, thus making processed foods less appealing. I promise! I used to live off of junk food, chocolate milk, minimal fresh fruits and veggies, and tons of bacon. Now the thought of eating any of that stuff makes me want to gag.

LEGUMES (BEANS, PEAS, AND LENTILS)

Why should you eat legumes? Legumes in general are high in protein, fiber, potassium, calcium, folic acid, iron, and many B vitamins. Practically all legumes support the kidneys and adrenals and regulate blood sugar and metabolism. They tend to have a low glycemic index, so they do not spike blood-sugar levels or promote weight gain. They are a healthy and safe carbohydrate for diabetics. So they're terrific for practically everyone, no matter what ails you. Remember when putting sprouts in your sandwich and on your salad became all the rage? It was for a good reason. Sprouted legumes and other plants, such as broccoli and radishes, are a great way to easily access their protein and other nutrients. Sprouting your beans also makes them easier to digest.

It's well known that legumes lower cholesterol and protect against heart disease. Their high fiber content aids in digestion, prevents constipation, and reduces the risk of colon cancer. Folic acid prevents birth defects. And the calcium content keeps your bones strong, unlike dairy. There are prebiotics in beans, which aid in beneficial bacteria growth in the intestine. Prebiotics are the precursor to probiotics and encourage their growth, and they also increase calcium absorption.

Worried about gas? This is the most common reason people use to avoid legumes. There are some simple tips to reduce the toots:

- Eat with fermented foods, such as sauerkraut, kimchee, coconut yogurt, and miso.

- Cook with fennel or cumin, kombu, ginger, fennel, kelp, or wakame to prevent gas.

- Soak for twelve hours in fresh grated ginger and plenty of water. This soaking process will also cause the beans to sprout, making minerals more available.

- Add a half teaspoon of the prebiotic source raw apple cider vinegar, a fermented food, during the last five to ten minutes of cooking.

- Chew well. Chewing helps break down the bean and stimulate saliva production, which further aids in digestion.

No need to get embarrassed every time you have a bean burrito anymore. So enjoy!

The list of legumes is endless. I've chosen some that are easy to find in most grocery stores, easy to cook, and are packed with nutrients and healing properties.

Black Beans

Black beans support the kidneys and reduce their associated emotional issues. They are high in folate, tryptophan, manganese, magnesium, vitamin B_1, iron, and phosphorus.

They nourish yin and blood, reduce low back pain, and stimulate urination. Black beans help treat infertility and impotence. Add them to chili or make your own burgers with them.

Cannellini Beans

Cannellini beans are high in iron (twice as much as beef), protein, magnesium, folate, and molybdenum. Molybdenum is a trace mineral that helps the body produce detoxifying enzymes. The beans help reduce lung issues and relieve grief and sadness. They're delicious in soups and tomato sauce.

Fava Beans

Fava beans nourish the spleen and reduce worry. They are high in iron, protein, folate, and riboflavin. They support digestion and act as a diuretic to reduce water retention. Make falafel with them or cook just like you would fresh green beans.

Garbanzo Beans/Chickpeas

Garbanzo beans support the stomach and heart and heal their associated emotions of worry and overthinking. They are high in unsaturated (healthy) fats, fiber, protein, iron, copper, phosphorus, tryptophan, and manganese. Chickpeas reduce the risk of cardiovascular disease, regulate blood sugar, and are high in antioxidants. What do I cook with chickpeas? Hummus, of course! But I also love them in curry and salads.

Green Beans

Green (or string) beans support the spleen and kidneys, treating the related emotions. They are high in vitamins K, C, B_3, and A, manganese, and folate. Green beans benefit the cardiovascular system, regulate blood sugar, and treat diarrhea. I like them raw as a snack. Or you can steam them for a couple of minutes and mix with your favorite spices.

Navy Beans

Navy beans support the lungs and issues around grief and sadness. They are high in folate, tryptophan, fiber, protein, iron, magnesium, vitamin B_1, copper, manganese, and phosphorous. They balance blood sugar, give you energy, and nourish the skin. These white beans are delicious in stews.

Kidney Beans

Kidney beans nourish the kidneys and reduce symptoms of anxiety and fear. They are high in folate, fiber, protein, manganese, iron, copper, vitamins B_1 and K, tryptophan, and phosphorus. Kidney beans reduce water retention and increase energy. The obvious choice is to put them in chili, but also try making a Caribbean classic—red beans and rice.

Lentils

Lentils support the kidneys, reducing fear and panic attacks. They are high in protein, iron, folate, fiber, vitamin B_1, potassium, manganese, copper, tryptophan, and molybdenum. They stimulate circulation and increase energy and strength.

Dal (an Indian soup) is my favorite way to eat lentils. You can also cook them, let them cool, and add them to any salad.

Lima Beans

Lima beans nourish the liver and lungs, treating the associated emotions. They are high in tryptophan, fiber, manganese, folate, protein, potassium, iron, copper, phosphorus, magnesium, and vitamin B_1. They benefit the skin, are very alkaline, and reduce the risk of heart disease.

I was never a fan of these nutrient-dense beans until I had them with snap peas, lemon, and mint. They're also perfect for minestrone.

Mung Beans

Mung beans are what I consider the king of beans. Originally from India and a staple of the cuisine, they help with almost any condition you can think of. I personally love them sprouted. It boosts their detoxification properties and gives better access to their nutrients. Mung beans support the liver and gallbladder, thus reducing anger and irritability. They are high in protein, phosphorus, potassium, calcium, fiber, magnesium, vitamins C and K, and folate. Their high fiber content helps reduce cholesterol. Mung beans also have isoflavones to regulate hormonal activity and are an excellent food choice for preventing osteoporosis. They are also a low glycemic index (diabetic-friendly) food.

Mung beans treat painful urination, heatstroke, water retention, food poisoning, dysentery, mumps, diarrhea, and burns, and they lower blood pressure.

I learned a delicious curry recipe with sprouted mung beans while staying with friends in Mumbai. It's really simple: curry powder, garlic, cayenne pepper, tomatoes, a little water or vegetable broth to cover, and mung beans. Simmer for fifteen minutes and eat.

Peas

Peas nourish the spleen and stomach and minimize worry and over-thinking. They are high in vitamins K, C, B_1, B_6, B_2, B_3, manganese, fiber, folate, tryptophan, phosphorus, protein, magnesium, copper, iron, zinc, and potassium. Peas are an anti-inflammatory, regulate blood sugar, and treat constipation, edema, burping, and coughing. There's nothing better than a big bowl of split pea soup on a cold day.

Soybeans

Soybeans strengthen the spleen and can reduce worry. They're high in protein, calcium, vitamins K and B_2, tryptophan, molybdenum, manganese, iron, phosphorus, fiber, magnesium, copper, and EFAs/omega-3s (healthy fats). Soybeans improve circulation, reduce blood pressure and cholesterol, moisten dryness, detoxify, improve vision, serve as a diuretic, lower fever, increase mother's milk, help with constipation, lessen skin problems, improve brain function, and help avoid toxemia during pregnancy. Edamame beans, which are

The Soy Controversy

Let me set the record straight: Organic soy is safe. I emphasize *organic* because in the United States most soy is genetically modified—93 percent, in fact. Abstain from soy found in processed foods labeled as hydrogenated oils, lecithin, emulsifiers, tocopherol (a vitamin E supplement), and/or proteins. If you're allergic, then avoid it. Otherwise, dig in.

Eat approximately three to five servings per day to get the most benefit. Women who eat soy regularly have a lower incidence of breast cancer. In Asia, where they eat soy daily, breast cancer rates are the lowest in the world—six times lower than in the United States. Guess who traditionally eats miso soup daily? Japanese women. When patients, friends, or family ask me about the safety of soy, especially in boys, I mention that there wouldn't be almost 1.5 billion people in China if the phytoestrogens in soy hurt boys' masculinity and hormones.

If you're worried about your thyroid, just make sure the soy is in its purest state— edamame, tempeh, or miso—and make sure you're getting enough iodine (found in sea vegetables, which also help prevent cancer): 150 to 1,000 micrograms a day.

immature green soybeans, are served at all Japanese restaurants. There's reason for this. This super-simple dish is tasty and great for you.

Black Soybeans

Black soybeans nourish the kidneys and treat fear and anxiety. They are high in protein, vitamins B_6 and K, calcium, iron, magnesium, phosphorus, potassium, and zinc. They improve circulation and detoxify, and they help with kidney disease, weak bones, and low back pain. Add them to tabbouleh to increase the health benefits.

Tofu

Tofu is high in iron, protein, copper, calcium, phosphorus, iron, selenium, manganese, magnesium, and potassium. It nourishes the spleen and stomach and supports the related emotions. It can reduce heart disease, inflammation, dry cough, fevers, and high blood pressure. If you have a weak spleen, make sure to cook it or add some ginger and garlic to your recipe. If you have any difficulties with digestion, tempeh (another form of fermented soy) is easier to digest than tofu. Use tofu in stir-fries, eggless egg salad, pudding, and in place of any meat in a recipe.

I can't believe I used to hate tofu. Now I can eat it plain right out of the package. It doesn't have much flavor, so use your creative cooking skills to spice it up. There are several companies also making marinated and flavored tofu.

Legumes have been a part of the human diet for thousands of years. There's a reason for that. We're meant to eat these nutrient-dense, fiber-rich foods. Make sure to incorporate them into your daily routine for better health and to balance the five elements of TCM.

WHOLE GRAINS

Carbs have gotten a bad rap since the early 1990s, but not all carbs are created equal. We need them for energy, and our bodies require them to operate. They are vital to brain function. Between 45 and 65 percent of your calories should come from carbohydrates. Just make sure to eat complex carbohydrates from whole grain sources. Choose brown rice over white rice and whole grain crackers over saltines.

Whole grains are a great source of nutrients and fiber. One of the more important benefits of whole grains is that they lower low-density lipoprotein (LDL, the bad cholesterol) and triglyceride levels, which contributes to an overall reduction in coronary heart disease risk factors. Over one-third of Americans have high LDL numbers, and they consume only 11 percent of their grains as whole grains. It's time to improve those numbers. Start by switching from refined grains to whole grains.

Ideally, you don't want to keep grains longer than six months, depending on the grain. They should have either no aroma or a slightly sweet smell; otherwise, they should not be purchased or eaten. Once grains and nuts, seeds, and oils have gone rancid, their nutrient content is reduced; they can cause an increased allergic reaction and sometimes can be toxic. So all those flours and grains you've had in the pantry for three years—it's time to toss them. You want to store uncooked grains in airtight glass containers in a cool, dry place. Freezing them will make them last usually up to twice as long.

Gluten

A lot of attention has been paid to gluten in recent years. You can refer to my sidebar on food allergies in chapter 9 to begin to see why gluten intolerance has become almost an epidemic. It's estimated that 5 to 10 percent of Americans have some level of sensitivity to gluten. Some studies put the number at more than 30 percent. Almost three million have celiac disease, an autoimmune disorder with potentially severe symptoms. Any exposure to gluten, even in minute doses, damages the lining of the small intestine. This leads to abdominal pain, gas, bloating, cramping, diarrhea, and malnourishment. The only known "cure" is complete avoidance of gluten.

If you have access, get grains, nuts, and spices in bulk. That way you can buy only what you need. One of my biggest pet peeves is wasting food. Americans throw away approximately 263 million pounds of mostly edible food every year. Buying in bulk is also a great way to save money, because bulk grains are always less expensive. Make sure to bring your own bags to reduce plastic use.

My list of whole grains includes some of the more popular and nutritious options. The mood-boosting benefits are high for all of them. For all the grains below, I cite which contain gluten and which don't.

Amaranth

Amaranth helps the lungs and the associated emotions. It is high in protein, vitamin C, fiber, magnesium, and calcium. Amaranth is gluten-free. Make a hot cereal with coconut milk, cinnamon, and your choice of fruit.

Storage
Pantry: 4 months
Freezer: 6 months

Barley

Barley strengthens the stomach and spleen and the related emotions. It is high in fiber, selenium, tryptophan, copper, manganese, and phosphorus. Barley has been shown to reduce cholesterol. It builds blood and yin. Barley reduces jaundice, inflammation, edema, fevers, and tumors. Pearled barley is a part of the Chinese herbal pharmacy and is included in most formulas designed to combat spleen deficiency and excess dampness. Barley contains gluten. Try the classic barley mushroom soup or use it in a gumbo.

Storage
Pantry: 6 months
Freezer: 1 year

Buckwheat

Buckwheat strengthens the stomach and heals the associated emotions. It is high in manganese, tryptophan, magnesium, phytonutrients (antioxidants), and fiber. Studies show that it reduces blood pressure and cholesterol and balances blood sugar. It strengthens blood vessels, stops chronic diarrhea and dysentery, reduces excessive sweating, and improves blood flow to the extremities. Buckwheat does not contain gluten. Buckwheat pancakes topped with blueberries are the perfect way to enjoy Sunday brunch.

Storage
Pantry: 2 months
Freezer: 4 months

Corn

Corn nourishes the spleen and stomach and alleviates worry. Corn is high in vitamins B_1 and B_5, fiber, vitamin C, antioxidants, phosphorus, folate, and manganese. It supports the heart, improves appetite, regulates digestion, reduces gallstones and edema, promotes dental health, and increases libido. Corn is gluten-free. Be careful to buy only organic corn, however, because most corn is genetically modified.

One of my fondest childhood memories is shucking fresh Silver Queen corn on the back porch and stuffing myself with several cobs every summer. I love corn on the cob so much that I don't add anything to it. No salt or butter needed. Or I chop it off raw and put it in salad. Corn chowder is another option for corn, especially when it's not in season and frozen is your only choice.

Storage
Pantry: 6 months
Freezer: 1 year

Millet

Millet strengthens the stomach, kidneys, and spleen and is used to treat worry and anxiety. It is high in manganese, tryptophan, magnesium, and phosphorus. It builds yin, relieves diabetes symptoms, gallstones, and indigestion, and reduces morning sickness. Pregnant women who are considered high risk should eat millet to help prevent a miscarriage. Millet is very alkaline and has strong antifungal properties. Millet is gluten-free. Substitute millet for rice in a pilaf, or combine the two.

Storage
Pantry: 2 months
Freezer: 4 months

Oats

Oats strengthen the spleen and reduce worry. They are high in manganese, selenium, tryptophan, phosphorus, vitamin B_1, fiber, magnesium, and protein. The high levels of phosphorus in oats support brain and nerve development in children. Oats build qi, remove cholesterol, and strengthen the heart and the immune system. They're great for dysentery, diabetes, hepatitis, bloating, and boils. Oats can be gluten-free or contain gluten, so read the label.

Did you say oatmeal cookies?!?! Yes, I know: I said I wouldn't put any desserts in the book, but I can't help myself. A better way to eat cooked oatmeal is to not add any sugar. Fruit will make it sweet enough.

Storage
Pantry: 4 months
Freezer: 8 months

Rice

Brown rice is great for strengthening the spleen and soothing the related emotions. Its high B-vitamin content relieves depression and anxiety. Brown rice is high in manganese, fiber, selenium, magnesium, tryptophan, and antioxidants. It reduces cholesterol, treats indigestion, and prevents gallstones. Brown rice is gluten-free.

Wild rice supports the kidneys and bladder and reduces the related emotions. It is high in protein, fiber, folate, vitamin B_6, magnesium, and manganese. Wild rice is gluten-free.

White rice is gluten-free but an inferior alternative to brown and wild rice. It is low in fiber because the husk and the bran are removed, which also means removing most of the nutrients found in unprocessed rice. White rice is higher in calories and can also spike blood sugar levels, increasing your risk of diabetes and weight gain. If you're in a rush to cook dinner, choose quinoa instead. It cooks just as quickly as white rice and is nutrient dense.

You can use rice in soups, stews, salads, or stir-fries.

Storage

Pantry: 6 months

Freezer: 1 year

Rye

Rye nourishes the spleen and stomach and treats the associated emotions. It is high in fiber, selenium, manganese, tryptophan, phosphorus, magnesium, and protein. It is a diuretic and aids in muscle, fingernail, hair, and bone growth. It reduces cholesterol, treats diabetes, and promotes digestive and cardiovascular health. Rye contains gluten. Rye bread with a tempeh Reuben sandwich is delicious.

Storage

Pantry: 6 months

Freezer: 1 year

Spelt

Spelt strengthens the spleen and reduces worry and overthinking. It is high in fiber, vitamin B_3, phosphorus, manganese, magnesium, protein, and copper. It aids in digestion, moistens dryness, and helps with diarrhea, constipation, and colitis. Spelt reduces the risk of cardiovascular disease. Spelt contains gluten. It can be used in breads, muffins, and crackers.

Storage

Pantry: 6 months

Freezer: 1 year

Whole Wheat

Wheat nourishes the kidneys, reduces fear and anxiety, and calms the mind. It helps with emotional instability and menopause symptoms. It is high in protein, fiber, manganese, niacin, iron, magnesium, and tryptophan. One cup of whole wheat contains 26 grams of protein. That's about half of what you need in a day. Wheat helps with inflammation, bloating and gas, bed-wetting, insomnia, and abnormal sweating, and it quenches thirst. Some sources say that wheat is more of a stomach and spleen tonic, which correlates with how it aids in digestion. Wheat contains gluten. Even if you're not allergic to gluten, be careful not to eat it too often. Overconsumption can lead to allergies.

I like wheat in the form of bulgur to make tabbouleh.

Storage

Pantry: 6 months

Freezer: 1 year

Now you can choose the most nourishing grains that will support you on your journey to total wellness. They'll increase your energy levels and keep you regular. Enjoy these mood boosters, and your spirits will soar.

NUTS AND SEEDS

Nuts and seeds are ideal as on-the-go snacks and added ingredients to many fortifying recipes. Craving something salty to munch on? Grab a handful of raw almonds instead of potato chips. A lot of dieters are worried about the fat content of nuts. Yes, they do contain fat, but they're mostly high in the good kind. If you're worried that they can make you gain weight, no need. Eat them in moderation and enjoy!

Nuts and seeds are a rich source of all important omega-3 essential fatty acids. Symptoms of a deficiency in omega-3s include infertility, fatigue, poor memory, lowered immunity, depression, heart disease, rheumatoid arthritis, and dry skin. Eating nuts, avocado, and algae can reduce inflammation, exercise-induced asthma, blood pressure, cholesterol, and joint pain. A handful of hemp seeds and walnuts will encourage weight loss, improve vision, and reduce your risk for heart disease and diabetes. Numerous studies have shown that different types of seeds and nuts can actually prevent weight gain, the development of heart disease, and the accumulation of LDL (bad) cholesterol. Nuts are a rich source of manganese, potassium, calcium, zinc, iron, magnesium, fluoride, B vitamins, and selenium.

Nuts also are high in vitamin E, which supports liver function and the related emotions. Vitamin E is required for maintaining the integrity of the cell membranes of mucous membranes and skin, thus protecting them from harmful oxygen free radicals. Want fewer wrinkles? Eat some guacamole or some almond butter on celery sticks.

In addition to vitamin E, seeds are high in fiber and monounsaturated fats that can help keep the heart healthy and the body disease-free. They are also great sources of protein, minerals, zinc, and other life-enhancing nutrients.

My storing tips for grains hold true for nuts and seeds as well.

Almonds
Almonds benefit the lungs and reduce grief and sadness. They are high in manganese, magnesium, tryptophan, copper, vitamin B_2, calcium, and phosphorus. Almonds prevent cardiovascular disease, treat asthma and coughing, regulate blood sugar, reduce LDL cholesterol, and eliminate free radicals. Try raw almond butter or milk, or thin almond slices in a salad.
Storage
Pantry: 9–12 months
Fridge: 1 year
Freezer: 2 years

Chia Seeds
Chia seeds are high in protein, fiber, calcium, phosphorus, manganese, and really high in omega-3s. They support the kidneys and reduce anxiety. Chia seeds relieve constipation, improve cardiovascular health, stabilize blood sugar, and help build muscle.

Chia seeds make a delicious pudding, similar to tapioca pudding but much better for you. Add them to your morning smoothie.
Storage
Pantry: 2–4 years
Fridge: 4 years

Flaxseeds

Flaxseeds nourish the spleen and relieve worry. They are high in omega-3 fatty acids, fiber, manganese, folate, magnesium, copper, phosphorus, and vitamin B_6. These seeds help to regulate hormones, act as a laxative; protect your heart; reduce blood pressure, pain, and inflammation; and strengthen the arteries. Sprinkle in your salad, or add to veggie burgers, fresh baked bread, or crackers.

Storage

UNGROUND

Pantry: 6–12 months

Freezer: 1 year

GROUND

Pantry: 1 week

Freezer: 1–2 months

Hazelnuts

These nuts are rich in dietary fiber, vitamins, and minerals, and packed with numerous health-promoting phytochemicals. They help protect from diseases and cancers. They are a rich source of manganese, potassium, calcium, copper, iron, B vitamins, magnesium, zinc, and selenium. Hazelnuts are the perfect addition to hot chocolate or tofu chocolate mousse. Chop some up in a butternut squash lasagna.

Storage

Pantry: 4–6 months

Fridge: 9 months

Freezer: 12 months

Hemp Seeds

Hemp seeds are over 30 percent protein and 40 percent fiber, and they are balanced with a three-to-one ratio of omega-6 to omega-3 oils. The Standard American Diet is very high in omega-6 and low in omega-3, which leads to inflammation, illness, and disease. Studies show that hemp seeds may prevent heart disease and many forms of cancer, as well as Alzheimer's and Parkinson's diseases. Add them to basil-based pesto or sprinkle on soup. Their flavor is very nutty.

Storage

Fridge or freezer: 8–12 weeks

Peanuts

Peanuts are actually legumes, but most people think they're nuts, so I put them in this section. Peanuts strengthen the spleen and are great for reducing worry and obsessive thinking. They are high in manganese, tryptophan, vitamin B_3, folate, copper, and protein. Peanuts promote heart health, reduce risk of stroke and colon cancer, increase breast milk and appetite, and relieve constipation. They provide over thirty essential nutrients and phytonutrients. Peanuts are a significant source of resveratrol, which is thought to reduce the risk of cardiovascular disease and cancer. They reduce edema and alleviate dry cough. Try them in an African stew with yams and tomatoes. My daily school lunch consisted of the classic peanut butter and jelly on white bread. Make a healthier version of it by switching to sprouted grain bread and unsweetened jam.

Storage
Pantry: 6–9 months
Fridge: 1 year
Freezer: 2 years

Pine Nuts

Pine nuts nourish the lungs and large intestines and treat all associated emotions. They are high in fiber, protein, iron, vitamins E and K, magnesium, phosphorus, potassium, zinc, copper, and manganese. Pine nuts relieve cough, dizziness, asthma, constipation, and rheumatism. Pine nuts are best known as an ingredient in pesto; I like them in many Italian dishes or a quinoa salad.

Storage
Pantry: 1–2 months
Fridge: 3–4 months
Freezer: 5–6 months

Pumpkin Seeds

Pumpkin seeds support the spleen and reduce worry and obsessive thinking. They are high in omega-3s, manganese, magnesium, phosphorus, tryptophan, copper, zinc, protein, vitamin K, and are a great source of iron. Pumpkin seeds are probably most well known as a treatment for a swollen prostate and prostate cancer. They reduce inflammation and arthritis, and are a diuretic. They can be added to salads or made into a delicious vegan-style pâté.

Storage
Pantry: 2–3 months
Fridge or freezer: 12 months

Quinoa

Quinoa is a seed, not a grain. It is native to the Andes of Bolivia, Chile, and Peru. Quinoa tonifies the kidneys and reduces fear and anxiety. Quinoa is a complete protein and has more calcium than milk. It is also high in iron, magnesium, tryptophan, healthy fats, copper, vitamin E, and phosphorus. Use it in a salad or hot cereal, or in place of rice.

Storage
Pantry or fridge: 1 year

Sesame Seeds

Black sesame seeds support the liver and kidneys and treat the emotions associated with both. They are high in calcium, copper, manganese, tryptophan, magnesium, iron, zinc, fiber, phosphorus, and vitamin B_1. They nourish yin and blood. Remember that tahini, which is found in hummus and makes a great addition to smoothies, is made from tan sesame seeds. I sprinkle black and tan sesame seeds on everything. They're extra delicious in curry, tofu steaks, and in peanut sauce over soba noodles.

Storage
Pantry: 3 months
Fridge: 9 months
Freezer: 1 year

Sunflower Seeds

Sunflower seeds help nourish the spleen and reduce worry. They are high in vitamins B_5, B_1, and E (90 percent of your daily requirement in one serving), manganese, magnesium, copper, tryptophan, selenium, phosphorus, and folate. Sunflower seeds are anti-inflammatory, lower cholesterol, improve heart health, increase energy, build muscle, and relieve constipation. Salad and homemade vegan cheese are two excellent ways to incorporate sunflower seeds.

Storage
Pantry: 2–3 months
Fridge and freezer: 1 year

Walnuts

Walnuts support the kidneys and reduce fear and anxiety. They are high in omega-3s, manganese, copper, tryptophan, and protein. They improve brain and adrenal function, help with short-term memory loss, reduce inflammation and pain, and increase fertility in men. Mix walnuts with tofu to make "meatballs" or sprinkle them on roasted brussels sprouts.

Storage
Pantry: 6 months
Fridge: 1 year
Freezer: 1–2 years

As you can see, nuts are fundamental to a healthy, happy you. They contain necessary nutrients for balanced hormones and optimal brain function. Whether it's depression or moodiness, these little bites of deliciousness improve your state of mind.

TUTTI FRUTTI

The old saying "An apple a day keeps the doctor away" is completely true. But the same could be said for most fruit. The health benefits are vast. They're high in fiber, vitamins, minerals, and antioxidants. Most fruits are anti-inflammatory and have cancer and other illness-fighting properties as well. Plus, when they're perfectly ripe, they taste so much better than any sugar-laden dessert. A friend of mine laughs at me because of the faces I make when I'm enjoying every bite of a plum in August. I'm in total bliss. You know that feeling? I truly don't need cake or chocolate if there's fresh fruit around.

Some of my patients are concerned about the sugar content in fruit. There's definitely some controversy about how much fruit is too much. I can say that, if there's access to other foods, it's rare for someone to eat too much fruit. Also, if you're going to choose between a candy bar and fruit salad, go for the fruit salad.

If you're at all concerned about weight issues or are a diabetic, some fruits have a lower glycemic index. Low glycemic foods don't spike blood-sugar levels, which is ideal to prevent weight gain, diabetes, and stress on the pancreas. Eating foods with high glycemic index values causes blood glucose levels to rise more rapidly, which results in greater insulin secretion by the pancreas, thus raising your risk of Type II diabetes. People who eat foods that have a low glycemic index tend to have a lower total body fat level.

There are studies showing that consuming high amounts of sugar, especially the high-fructose corn syrup found in soda and many processed foods, can increase your risk of pancreatic cancer. Pancreatic cancer is considered one of the hardest to treat, because once you have symptoms and it's detected, it's usually too far gone to heal.

Eating low glycemic fruits means you won't spike your blood sugar levels and have an energy crash later that could make you cranky or tired. Lower glycemic index fruits include blackberries, strawberries, blueberries, cranberries, raspberries, cherries, peaches, pears, grapefruit, apples, kiwi, limes, lemons, and pomegranates.

If you're diabetic, discuss your fruit intake with a qualified nutritionist. If you have a Candida overgrowth of yeast in the body, you should avoid fruit until you've treated it. With all of advantages of eating fruit, however, there are few tips to keep in mind. When consuming a diet high in fat and/or protein, your body can't metabolize fruit and absorb its mood-boosting nutrients very well. Eating fruit by itself or in a green salad will optimize the health benefits of your meal.

I think fruits are best eaten fresh and on their own. Juicing and putting them in smoothies are two of my favorite ways to enjoy fruit.

Every morning I start my day with a large glass of lemon water to hydrate, alkalinize my body to prevent any illness or inflammation, get a dose of vitamin C, and wake up my digestion. Next I get out my Vitamix and blend up a delicious, fortifying breakfast: unsweetened hemp milk, chia and flaxseeds, carrots, kale, spinach, banana, apple or orange, mango, and whatever frozen berries I have in the fridge. This keeps me energized for hours.

Ideally, you want to eat your fruits and veggies in season. They have higher nutrient content and taste much better. We're not meant to eat fresh raspberries that were grown halfway around the world in the middle of winter. There are many reasons to eat locally as much as possible. Local, family-owned farms are more likely to be conservative in their use of toxic chemicals, so if you can't buy from an organic farm, small nonorganic farms are the next best choice. Small farms are also more likely to sell their crops when they're at their peak, so you get the tastiest and freshest of the bunch. Eating local is better for the environment: If your pears are coming from another state or even another country, they have a long way to travel, and with that comes gas for transportation and an increased carbon footprint. Last but not least, supporting your local farmers and family businesses builds the local economy and community.

Frozen is the next best option to fresh, especially if you live in a place that doesn't have good access to recently picked produce. Frozen fruits and vegetables tend to be harvested right at the peak of ripeness. They're almost immediately frozen, which helps retain their nutritional content. Research now suggests that frozen often is better than fresh, because it can take days for your blueberries to arrive at your grocery store. Every day after those blueberries have been picked, they quickly start to lose essential vitamins and minerals.

I've chosen each of these fruits because of their incredible health-stimulating benefits and their accessibility.

Apples

Apples nourish the spleen and can reduce worry. They are a good source of fiber, vitamins C, K, and B_6, riboflavin, and thiamin. Apples can remove cholesterol, heavy metals, and even radiation from the body. They stimulate digestion, balance blood sugar levels, and reduce blood pressure.

Season: Late summer through fall; keep in cold storage until spring.

Raw Apple Cider Vinegar

Raw apple cider vinegar can benefit you so much more than just helping with liver symptoms. I recommend drinking it daily to almost all my patients.

First off, it's highly alkaline in nature. I know, it seems counterintuitive that a vinegar would be alkaline instead of highly acidic. This is how your body processes it, not how it tastes. Consuming more alkaline foods reduces inflammation and risk of disease, and aids in digestion.

Apple cider vinegar is high in calcium and potassium. It can help eliminate viruses, bacteria, and fungus. It can prevent a spike in glucose after meals and heartburn. It helps regulate blood pressure and reduce cholesterol. Apple cider vinegar treats constipation and can heal problem skin. It's also a prebiotic, which helps your body nourish the healthy gut flora in your digestive tract and increases its health benefits.

The taste is really strong, so I would recommend diluting 2 tablespoons with some water. If you still can't handle the taste, a drop of liquid Stevia should sweeten it right up. I like to drink apple cider vinegar in just a small amount of water, like doing a shot. Some people prefer diluting 2 tablespoons in a gallon of water and drinking it throughout the day.

Apricots

Apricots support the lungs and relieve dehydration, asthma, cough, anemia, and nourish yin. They will help you with grief and sadness. Apricots are a good source of beta-carotene, fiber, copper, potassium, cobalt, and vitamins A and C.

Season: Late spring through early summer

Avocados

Avocados nourish the spleen, blood, and yin. They support emotions related to the spleen. They relieve constipation and treat anemia. Avocados are high in monounsaturated fat, fiber, vitamins C and K, and folate.

Season: Year-round

Bananas

Bananas benefit the Metal element and help with grief and letting go. They are very high in potassium, fiber, vitamins C and B_6, and manganese. As an added bonus, they are a natural antacid. Potassium is an essential mineral that helps balance your sodium levels to keep your blood pressure from getting too high. It also plays a role in heart, muscle, and digestive function. Bananas clear heat, lubricate

Wine

I get asked a lot about wine. Is it really that healthy? Occasionally having a glass or two of organic, sulfite-free wine is fine. It can thin the blood and help you decompress after a long day. But it's better to eat the right foods, so you don't have plaque buildup in your arteries or high cholesterol in the first place. The pesticides, sulfites, alcohol, and sugar content aren't great for you. But I'm all about taking pleasure in what you eat so you don't feel deprived. Most markets carry some organic options. If you're new to veganism, many wines aren't vegan, so double-check before purchasing.

lungs and intestines (for constipation), and lower blood pressure. They also help with ulcers, hemorrhoids, dry cough, and colitis.

Since they're so incredibly good for you, bananas are the one fruit I always include in my morning smoothie.

Season: Year-round

Cherries

Cherries nourish the spleen and reduce worry. They are high in iron, so they're good for anemia. They're also high in fiber, copper, and manganese, and are a very good source of vitamins A and C. Cherries treat arthritis, dysentery, male sexual dysfunction, diarrhea, measles, gout, and rheumatism. They also benefit the skin, stimulate appetite, and quench thirst.

Season: Late spring and summer

Grapefruit

Grapefruit supports the spleen and stomach and treats worry and overthinking. It is high in vitamin C, fiber, and potassium. It reduces fevers, is highly alkaline, stimulates digestion, circulates qi, and detoxifies alcohol intoxication. Grapefruit improves appetite and reduces dry cough.

Season: Fall through late spring

Grapes

Grapes support the stomach and spleen and the related emotions. They are high in vitamin K and manganese. Grapes nourish qi and blood, reduce fatigue and edema, and help with painful urination, hepatitis, arthritis and tendonitis, anemia, flu symptoms, jaundice, and irritability.

Season: Late summer into early fall

Lemons

Lemons are a good source of folate, potassium, and vitamin C. An added bonus to consuming lemons and other food that have high levels of vitamin C is that C prevents bruising and keeps your skin young and supple. Lemons are very alkaline in nature. They nourish the spleen, reduce worry, stimulate metabolism, and aid digestion. Make sure to have lemons if you're experiencing any of the following: dysentery, colds and flu, phlegm buildup, edema, high blood pressure, diabetes, or gas. They nourish yin, aid in the absorption of water, reduce inflammation, and help rid the body of toxins. They are also a natural antibiotic. So add lemon to your water when you're fighting a cold or are around someone who is sick.

Season: Winter through spring

Mangoes

Mangoes strengthen the stomach and reduce worry. They are high in fiber and vitamin B_6, and a very good source of vitamins A and C. They regenerate body fluids if you're dehydrated, stop coughs, aid digestion, and shrink an enlarged prostate.

Season: Summer

Oranges

Oranges support the spleen and stomach and their related emotions. They are an excellent source of thiamin, folate, potassium, and vitamin C. They reduce inflammation and arthritis, boost immunity, lubricate lungs, eliminate mucus, increase appetite, and quench thirst.

Season: Winter and spring

Peaches

Peaches moisten a dry cough, treat constipation, and reduce high blood pressure. They support the functions of the large intestine and stomach and aid in letting go and worry. They are high in fiber, vitamins A and C, niacin, and potassium.

Season: Summer

Pears

Pears treat the lungs and grief. They are high in vitamins C and K, and fiber. Pears are excellent for helping with any lung condition, including loss of voice, asthma, and coughing (especially dry cough, but also to reduce phlegm). They regenerate body fluids, quench thirst, calm the heart, relieve restlessness and constipation, promote urination, and detoxify the body. They also help with lesions and alcohol intoxication.

Season: Fall

Pineapple

Pineapple is great for sunstroke, anorexia, diarrhea, edema, and thirst. It also serves as a diuretic. It is high in fiber, thiamin, vitamins B_6 and C, copper, and manganese. Pineapple clears heat, aids digestion, reduces thirst and irritability, and stops diarrhea.

Season: Spring through early summer

Pomegranates

Pomegranates nourish the heart and relieve the associated emotions. They are high in fiber, folate, and vitamins C and K. Pomegranates build blood, treat anemia, combat intestinal worms and canker sores, and detoxify the liver.

Season: Fall

Raspberries

Raspberries strengthen the liver and kidneys and their associated emotions. They are high in vitamins C and K, iron, magnesium, fiber, and manganese. Raspberries treat anemia, promote labor, and regulate the menstrual cycle.

Season: Summer

Strawberries

Strawberries strengthen the spleen and reduce worry. They are a good source of vitamin C, folate, potassium, fiber, and manganese. They lubricate the lungs, promote body fluids, and counteract alcohol intoxication. They help with dry cough and dry/sore throat, increase appetite, nourish yin, aid in digestion, and relieve painful urination.

Season: Spring through summer

Watermelon

Watermelon nourishes the spleen and treats worry. It is high in potassium and vitamins A and C. It reduces fever, treats constipation, urinary tract infections, edema, canker sores, and depression, quenches thirst, relieves irritability, and helps with sunstroke problems, edema, jaundice, detoxification, and difficult urination.

Season: Summer

You can eat delicious, health-promoting fruit throughout the year. If you're the type to forget about grabbing an apple to take to work or hate all that washing, chopping, and cleanup, then buy organic frozen fruit. Fresh, local, and in season is always best, but frozen is way better than none at all.

EAT YOUR VEGGIES

Vegetables. Why are we raised to think eating our veggies is a punishment? We should really be taught how lucky we are to be able to enjoy these colorful, fortifying, tasty treats. Who wants to put food coloring, corn syrup, steroids, and hydrogenated fats into our young, naturally energetic bodies? These "foods" just slow us down—mentally, physically, and emotionally. Do you remember being so proud to get the highest grade on a test? Or being the fastest runner in gym class? Well, fresh whole foods support those successes. They give you brainpower and muscle strength. Lucky Charms and Cheetos do not. And the best part is that you can indulge in vegetables without any guilt. You can eat pretty much all the vegetables you want. All of them are packed full of nutrients, antioxidants, disease-fighting properties, fiber, and tons of flavor.

If you have a bunch of vegetables and don't know what to do with them, try making a soup. They're pretty easy to make, and they can be soothing and cozy. Plus, they taste *soooo* good. During the winter, there's nothing better. If you have children, soups are the best way to sneak in vegetables. Throw them in a pot with some vegetable broth and a couple of spices for less than an hour, and you'll have a delicious meal.

Like fruit, vegetables should ideally be eaten in season and from local providers to get the most out of them.

Alfalfa Sprouts

Alfalfa sprouts benefit spleen and stomach and the related emotions. They treat constipation, edema, eczema, and rashes. Alfalfa sprouts are an excellent source of protein (4 grams per 100-gram serving); vitamins A, C, and K, thiamin, calcium, iron, fiber, riboflavin, folate, magnesium, phosphorus, zinc, copper, and manganese. The obvious choices for alfalfa sprouts are on a sandwich or in a salad.

Season: Year-round

Asparagus

Asparagus supports the kidneys and reduces fear and anxiety. It is high in vitamins K, B_1, B_2, B_3, B_6, C, and A, folate, tryptophan, manganese, fiber, copper, phosphorus, and protein. It has anti-inflammatory and antioxidant benefits. Asparagus regulates blood sugar, improves heart health, reduces cholesterol and high blood pressure, and helps with dry cough. It encourages healthy bacterial growth in the digestive tract. I love it in creamy asparagus soup or steamed with lemon and garlic.

Season: Spring

Beets

Beets calm the heart and anxiety. They are high in folate, iron, potassium, fiber, manganese, vitamin C, magnesium, and tryptophan. They purify the blood and liver, reduce inflammation, and relieve constipation. Beets also alleviate anemia and herpes outbreaks. Beets in a juice with carrot, apple, celery, and ginger are an excellent immune booster and pick-me-up. You can add one beet to carrot-ginger soup for added flavor and nutrients.

Beets are great for nourishing yin (the calming aspect of one's health) and the heart in Chinese nutrition. So if you're experiencing yin-deficiency symptoms discussed further in Part II, such as menopause or trouble sleeping, add some beets to your morning juice, lunchtime salad, or carrot-ginger soup. You'll soon be sleeping like a baby. Another benefit of beets is great poops. A beet a day will keep things moving. And when you're stopped up, you're definitely going to be cranky.

Season: Year-round

Bell Peppers

Bell peppers strengthen the stomach and reduce worry. Red bell pepper strengthens the heart. They improve appetite, promote blood circulation, and reduce edema. Bell peppers are chock-full of vitamin C, K, and B_6. They are also a good source of thiamin, niacin, folate, magnesium, copper, fiber, potassium, and manganese. I love red bell pepper on its own. Whenever I cook with them, I end up eating half before they make it into my dish. It adds a nice flavor and crunchy texture to chili if you put it in for just a few minutes at the end of cooking.

Season: Summer and early fall

Cabbage

Cabbage nourishes the stomach and relieves overthinking and worry. It also relieves depression and irritability. It is high in vitamins C, K, B_1, B_2, and B_6, fiber, iodine, manganese, and omega-3s. The outer leaves are high in vitamin E. Cabbage is a cancer fighter, aids digestion (especially when raw and fermented), reduces inflammation, and helps with hot flashes, constipation, colds, parasites, and ulcers. Maybe it's my German heritage, but I love sauerkraut. I eat it by itself and mix it in where you wouldn't expect. I drop a bunch of it on top of my stir-fry.

Season: Best in late fall and winter, but available year-round

Carrots

Carrots are great for supporting the spleen and its related emotions. One serving contains over 600 percent of your daily requirements for vitamin A. This is what makes them such a powerhouse against cancer, ear infections, vision problems, and inflammation, and in improving skin conditions.

They are also high in vitamins K, C, B_6, B_1, and B_3, fiber, potassium, and manganese. Carrots improve liver function, nourish yin, dissolve stones and tumors, treat acne, kill some parasites, help with urinary tract infections and dysentery, increase mother's milk, and aid in calcium metabolism. Carrots are delicious in juices, salads, soups, and stews. Have carrot sticks around at all times for a healthy snack.

Season: Year-round

Cauliflower

Cauliflower strengthens the spleen and reduces worry. It is a good source of vitamins C, K, and B$_6$, thiamin, riboflavin, niacin, magnesium, phosphorus, fiber, folate, pantothenic acid, potassium, and manganese. Cauliflower treats constipation and weakened digestion. Mix some in with your mashed potatoes or in pad thai. I'm addicted to the buffalo-style cauliflower at a nearby restaurant.

Season: Best in late fall and winter, but available year-round

Celery

Celery supports the stomach and spleen and reduces worry as well as anger; nourishes connective tissue; reduces inflammation, fevers, and high blood pressure; and promotes sweating. It is also a good choice for those suffering from rheumatism, diabetes, vertigo, nervousness, burning urination, or canker sores. Celery sticks with hummus or almond butter are an excellent snack or addition to your lunch. Mix them in with garbanzo beans and Vegenaise for a mock tuna salad.

Season: Best in late fall and winter, but available year-round

Cucumbers

Cucumbers are a great veggie for nourishing the spleen and stomach. So when you're the type who can't turn off your head, add some to your salad and daily green juice. Cucumber skin is high in silicon and chlorophyll, so don't peel it. Cucumbers are also high in vitamins A, C, and K, pantothenic acid, magnesium, phosphorus, manganese, and potassium. They are a diuretic, eliminate toxins, reduce inflammation, quench thirst, purify skin, relieve jaundice, dry cough, and edema, cool burns, and treat heat stroke. Nothing makes me happier than to eat fresh cucumber and heirloom tomatoes with a touch of lemon juice in the summer.

Season: Summer

Eggplant

Eggplant also supports the spleen and stomach and their related emotions. It is high in phytonutrients and antioxidants. It is also a good source of vitamins C and K, thiamin, niacin, vitamin B$_6$, pantothenic acid, magnesium, phosphorus, copper, fiber, folate, potassium, and manganese. Eggplant supports brain function, protects the heart and blood vessels, and reduces cholesterol and blood pressure. It can remove blood clots and shrink tumors. Eggplant in lasagna or almost any pasta dish is divine.

Season: Summer through early fall

Kale

Kale supports the stomach and its emotions. It is high in chlorophyll, iron, calcium, vitamins A, K, C, and B_6, manganese, fiber, folate, protein, thiamin, riboflavin, magnesium, phosphorus, and copper. It aids digestion, heals ulcers, reduces inflammation, prevents cancer, detoxifies the liver, and supports heart health. My favorite way to have kale is in a salad with a lot of different vegetables. Juicing it with other greens and lemon will give you a better energy boost than a cup of coffee.

Season: Best in fall and winter

Leeks

Leeks support the liver and reduce anger and irritability. They are high in fiber, vitamin B_6, iron and magnesium, vitamins A, C, and K, folate, and manganese. Leeks' high antioxidant content protects the heart and blood vessels, and they also treat diarrhea. Leeks in lentil soup—there's nothing else like it.

Season: Fall through spring

Lettuce

Lettuce acts as a sedative to reduce anxiety. Iceberg lettuce supports the stomach and large intestines and aids in letting go and turning off the mind. Depending on the type of lettuce, it can be high in chlorophyll, iron, vitamins A, K, and C, folate, manganese, chromium, and potassium. Even iceberg lettuce is a good source of nutrients. It's high in thiamin, vitamins A, C, K, and B_6, iron, potassium, fiber, folate, and manganese. It reduces edema, increases breast milk, supports the heart, and treats hemorrhoids and blood in urine.

Season: Best in spring, but available year-round

Mushrooms

Mushrooms are used medicinally quite a bit in Chinese medicine, especially reishi mushrooms. Shiitake mushrooms support the stomach and its related emotions. Black mushrooms nourish the kidneys and reduce anxiety. They are high in vitamins B_3, B_2, B_5, and B_6, manganese, phosphorus, fiber, potassium, and selenium. Because of their high levels of interferon, some mushrooms are incredibly powerful at strengthening your immunity and preventing cancer. They also can reduce hypertension and cholesterol levels. Add to veggie burgers, stir-fries, and stuffed bell peppers.

Season: Year-round, if cultivated

Onions

Onions support the lungs and their related emotions. They are high in chromium, vitamins C and B_6, fiber, manganese, molybdenum, and tryptophan. They can reduce blood clots and cholesterol, remove heavy metals, lower blood pressure, kill some parasites, improve the metabolism of protein, and inhibit viral, fungal, and yeast growth. Onions improve bone density and are anti-inflammatory. Finely chopped onions can add flavor to almost any dish. I like to put them in chili and curry.

Season: Spring through fall

Parsley Leaf

Parsley is that little green sprig most restaurants add for decoration, but you really should eat it. Parsley is high in iron, vitamins A, C, and K, chlorophyll, calcium, and magnesium. It protects against rheumatoid arthritis, heart disease, and cancer. It increases energy and digestion, acts as a diuretic, and benefits the adrenal glands. Mix it in with tabbouleh, your green juice, and pesto sauce.

Season: Year-round

Parsnips

Parsnips support the spleen and stomach and their related emotions. They are high in fiber, vitamin C, folate, and magnesium. Parsnips clean out the liver, gallbladder, and intestines. They strengthen the immune system and can reduce coughs. Parsnips are delicious in lentil soup, mixed in with mashed potatoes, or roasted with carrots and beets.

Season: Fall through spring

Potatoes

Potatoes nourish the spleen and stomach and their related emotions. They are high in potassium, protein, vitamin C, iron, fiber (with the skin), vitamin B_6, thiamin, niacin, folate, phosphorus, and manganese. Potatoes aid in digestion and constipation, relieve arthritis and rheumatism, reduce inflammation, lower blood pressure and ulcers, and relieve eczema. And like all root vegetables, they nourish yin.

Potatoes are traditionally found in samosas and curry. And how about that other wonderful tradition, the baked potato?

Season: Late summer and early fall

Pumpkin

Pumpkin is one of my all-time favorite vegetables, so I want to highlight it. It's high in all of the following:

FIBER
- Reduces bad cholesterol levels, thus reducing the risk of heart disease
- Controls blood sugar levels
- Promotes healthy digestion
- Encourages weight loss

POTASSIUM
- Balances fluid levels
- Promotes strong bones
- Necessary for energy production
- Maintains healthy blood pressure

ALPHA-CAROTENE AND BETA-CAROTENE
- Improves vision and reduces risk of cataracts
- Reverses sun damage to the skin and slows the aging process
- Is an anti-inflammatory
- Prevents tumor growth
- Boosts the immune system
- Protects against heart disease

VITAMIN C
- Boosts immunity
- Reduces high blood pressure and heart disease
- Regulates cholesterol levels

VITAMIN E
- Slows aging by protecting the skin from sun damage
- Reduces the risk of Alzheimer's disease and certain cancers

MAGNESIUM
- Promotes a strong immune system
- Strengthens the bones
- Supports heart function

PANTOTHENIC ACID/VITAMIN B_5
- Balances hormone levels
- Manages stress levels

Season: Fall

Spinach

Spinach nourishes the spleen and helps with its emotions. It is high in vitamins K, A, C, B_2, B_1, B_6, and E, manganese, folate, magnesium, iron, calcium, potassium, antioxidants, tryptophan, fiber, copper, and protein. Spinach is anti-inflammatory, prevents prostate cancer and osteoporosis, detoxifies the blood, and relieves constipation. I put spinach in my morning smoothie, tomato sauce, pesto, and salads. You name it, it's got spinach in it.

Season: Year-round

Sweet Potatoes

Sweet potatoes benefit the spleen and stomach and their emotions. They are high in vitamins A, C, and B_6, manganese, copper, fiber, and potassium. They are high in antioxidants, are anti-inflammatory, nourish yin to reduce menopausal symptoms, increase breast milk, and balance blood sugar for diabetics. They treat diarrhea and constipation, jaundice, edema, ascites, night blindness, and breast abscesses.

Season: Fall and winter

Swiss Chard

Swiss chard clears heat, detoxifies, and nourishes blood in cases of anemia. It is a good source of thiamin, folate, zinc, fiber, vitamins A, C, B₂ (riboflavin), B₆, E, and K, calcium, iron, magnesium, phosphorus, potassium, copper, and manganese. I eat swiss chard in soup with cannellini beans and in salad, or I sauté it with some tomatoes, garlic, and garbanzo beans.

Season: Summer

Tomatoes

Tomatoes are actually a fruit, but people think of them as a vegetable. They support the stomach and address worry and overthinking. They are high in vitamins C, A, and K, molybdenum, and potassium. Tomatoes aid in digestion, nourish yin, and reduce high blood pressure, gout, and rheumatism.

When they're perfectly ripe, tomatoes can be eaten on their own—there's nothing plain about them. I also love them in tomato sauce that's quick and simple to make. Use garlic, onions, fresh basil, whole peeled tomatoes, and a little oregano. Let this simmer for at least an hour. The next day it always tastes better. You can also add some of your favorite vegetables to it, like eggplant, zucchini, yellow squash, or mushrooms.

Season: Summer

Listen to your mother and eat your vegetables. Two-thirds of your plate should be vegetables. Find the ones you love. Get creative and try new ones every week or every month. Take a cooking class or buy a new cookbook to get inspired. Have friends over for dinner regularly to try out your new creations.

For easy access, I've grouped all the emotions and relevant foods mentioned throughout the book into one section. This way you can look up your feeling that day or week and know what to buy at that market or grab out of the fridge. If it's PMS time of the month, check out the anger foods. Going through a breakup? Go to the section on heartbreak. Feeling a little bit of everything? Make a yummy, soul-soothing soup with ingredients from each section.

Fear and Anxiety

Symptoms	TCM diagnosis	Foods to eat	Foods to minimize
general fear and anxiety	kidney qi deficiency	grapes, plums, boysenberries, celery, turnips, walnuts, string beans, whole wheat, watercress, asparagus, millet, endive, cabbage, black beans, amaranth, rye, barley, quinoa, oats, kelp, nori, chlorella, miso, tangerine, plums, cinnamon, dill seed, and chive	caffeine, soda, and stimulants
insomnia, night sweats, anxiety, dryness, symptoms worse at night	kidney yin deficiency	beets, carrots, yams, radish, chlorella, kelp, spirulina, chica seeds, black sesame seeds, quinoa, radish, wild rice, sweet potatoes, mung beans, kidney beans, black beans, soybeans, string beans, watermelon, blueberries, blackberries, raspberries, and aloe vera gel	onions, leeks, basil, horseradish, cayenne, spicy peppers, ginger, cloves, and cinnamon
low back pain, coldness, diarrhea; symptoms often are worse in morning	kidney yang deficiency	walnuts, black beans, quinoa, ginger, cloves, cinnamon, leeks, fennel, lentils, and anise	raw foods, iced drinks, and fruit

Anger

Symptoms	TCM diagnosis	Foods to eat	Foods to minimize
general feeling of anger		lima beans, raspberries, celery, and leeks	
PMS symptoms, flank (sides of torso) pain, holding onto resentment and anger, easily angered	stagnation of qi in the liver	beets, mustard greens, turnip, cabbage, cauliflower, broccoli, quinoa, asparagus, rye, romaine lettuce, alfalfa, pine nuts, brussels sprouts, vinegars (brown rice, rice wine, apple cider), dill, cumin, fennel, black pepper, marjoram, ginger, cardamom, onion, basil, mint, turmeric, bay leaf, horseradish, strawberries, peaches, and cherries	spicy food
concern over toxins in food, water, air, clothing, and beauty products	liver toxicity	cucumber, mung beans, tofu, millet, plums, radish, rhubarb, daikon radish, spirulina, lettuce, kelp, nori, kombu, wakame, chlorella, parsley, kale, collard greens, and sprouts (alfalfa, sunflower, clover, mung, broccoli, bean)	sugar, alcohol, coffee, processed food, food coloring, food additives, and pesticides

Anger (continued)

Symptoms	TCM diagnosis	Foods to eat	Foods to minimize
menopause, hot flashes, night sweats, insomnia, hot hands and feet, dry mouth, and/or any chemotherapy side effects	not of enough yin in your liver	parsley, artichoke, carrots, avocado, lemon, lime, mulberries, yams, parsnips, hemp and flax seed, mung beans, and aloe vera gel	onions, leeks, basil, horseradish, cayenne, spicy peppers, ginger, cloves, and cinnamon
symptoms of anemia: light-headedness, muscle cramps, leg cramps, fatigue, pale nail bed, shortness of breath, and poor concentration	liver blood deficiency	blackstrap molasses, soybeans, lentils, spinach, collard greens, blackberries, raspberries, prunes, and grapes	coffee, sweets, and iced drinks
neurological issues such as Parkinson's, multiple sclerosis, epilepsy, tremors, stroke, and seizures	"liver wind"	celery, oats, flaxseeds, black soybeans, pine nuts, black sesame seeds, basil, sage, fennel, anise, peppermint, chamomile, coconut, ginger, and strawberries	white flour, white rice, animal fats, and processed foods

Heartache, Sadness, and Shock

Symptoms	TCM diagnosis	Foods to eat	Foods to minimize
emotional and physical heart complaints	heart imbalance	corn, shiitake mushrooms, whole wheat, brown rice, green beans, peanuts, pears, oats, garbanzo beans, beets, mulberries, lemon, pomegranate, dill, basil, chamomile, marjoram, bell peppers, celery, lettuce, romaine lettuce, cucumbers (with skin), and tomatoes	caffeine, onions, and garlic
palpitations on exertion, fatigue, muscle weakness, sweating without exertion, and lowered heart rate while exercising	heart qi deficiency; overexercising is one of the main causes	cinnamon, carrots, daikon radishes, red radishes, saffron, onions, garlic, chick peas, pomegranate, and cherries	oranges, almonds, cashews, peanuts, wheat, tangerines, and spinach
palpitations, cold limbs or feeling cold, fatigue, and spontaneous sweating	heart yang deficiency	qi-fortifying foods listed above (cinnamon, carrots, daikon radishes, red radishes, saffron, onions, garlic, and cherries), plus walnuts, chives, cayenne pepper, raspberries, strawberries, blueberries, blackberries, ginger, clove, and cardamom	alfalfa sprouts, mangoes, banana, and iced drinks

Symptoms	TCM diagnosis	Foods to eat	Foods to minimize
palpitations, insomnia, nightmares, anxiety, startling easily, dizziness, pale lips/complexion, poor long-term memory, and inability to concentrate	heart blood deficiency—not enough healthy blood flowing through the heart	yams, sweet potatoes, parsnips, turnips, pumpkin, millet, spelt, beets, cherries, grapes, butternut squash, beets, onions, leeks, garlic, parsley, chard, kale, and bok choy	caffeine, sweets, and iced drinks
night sweats, hot flashes, palpitations, insomnia, nightmares, anxiety, startling easily, dry mouth, and poor long-term memory	heart yin deficiency	fava, mung, and kidney beans, persimmons, apples, beets, black sesame seeds, flaxseeds, seaweed, peaches, blueberries, blackberries, mangoes, bananas, coconut, endive, and asparagus	coffee, vinegar, garlic, leeks, sonions, basil, horseradish, cayenne, spicy peppers, ginger, cloves, and cinnamon
palpitations, mental illnesses, thirst, red face, bitter taste in mouth in morning, dark urine, phlegm, insomnia, nightmares, restlessness, and manic behavior	heart phlegm	kale, collard greens, mustard greens, ginger, seaweed, barley, and bamboo shoots	nuts, seeds, dairy, and grains

Worry and Overthinking

Symptoms	TCM diagnosis	Foods to eat	Foods to minimize
slow metabolism, varicose veins, premature sagging of skin, gas, bloating, loose stool or constipation, bruising easily, craves sugar, hernias, and hypothyroid symptoms—gains weight easily, runs cold, hair loss	spleen qi deficiency	millet, corn, carrots, cabbage, celery, spinach, peanuts, mango, oranges, grapes, cherries, spelt, pumpkin seeds, sunflower seeds, cauliflower, rye, garbanzo beans, soybeans, squash, potatoes, string beans, yams, tofu, sweet potatoes, brown rice, amaranth, peas, chestnuts, apricots, and cantaloupe, oats, rice (brown or red) spelt, flax seedsparsnips, shiitake mushrooms, eggplant, apples, squash, turnip, carrots, parsnips, black beans, peas, sweet potato, yam, pumpkin, garbanzo beans, leeks, ginger, garlic, fennel, black pepper, onion, nutmeg, and cinnamon	wheat, seaweeds, raw veggies and fruit, dairy, sugar or sweetened foods, tofu, sprouts, and spinach
water retention, edema, diarrhea, facial swelling	spleen qi deficiency with damp	barley, rye, corn, celery, lettuce, scallions, ginger, garlic, grapefruit, alfalfa sprouts, radish, millet, fava beans, and adzuki beans	same as above

Grief, Sadness, and Letting Go

Symptoms	TCM diagnosis	Foods to eat	Foods to minimize
runny nose, coughing up mucus, sinus congestion or infection	excess phlegm in the lungs	kelp, turnips, fennel, flaxseeds, cayenne pepper, onions, pears, watercress, garlic, ginger, mushrooms, and papaya	dairy, yeast, wheat, soy, peanuts, and sugar
shortness of breath on the exhale, coughing, easily catches colds and flus, fatigue, asthma	lung qi deficiency	rice, oats, carrots, almonds, mustard greens, banana, pears, amaranth, pine nuts, sweet potatoes, cannelini beans, yam, navy beans, potato, ginger, kale, sweet potato, carrots, spinach, turnip greens, collard greens, butternut squash, winter squash, romaine lettuce, cabbage, beet greens, coriander, basil, parsley, garlic, blackstrap molasses, and lima beans	tofu, seaweeds, and iced drinks
when dry weather affects your lungs and breathing or aggravates your symptoms	dryness in lungs	nori, almonds, pine nuts, peanuts, sesame seeds, soybeans, tofu, tempeh, soy milk, spinach, barley, millet, pear, apple, persimmon, barley malt, and rice syrup	barley, rye, corn, celery, lettuce, scallions, ginger, garlic, and radish

Grief, Sadness, and Letting Go *(continued)*

Symptoms	TCM diagnosis	Foods to eat	Foods to minimize
coughing up green or yellow phlegm, burning sensation when coughing, pneumonia, or bronchitis (smokers always have excess heat in their lungs)	heat in the lungs	cabbage, asparagus, bamboo shoots, banana, pears, oranges, lemon, watercress, cauliflower, apples, carrots, lime, bok choy, cantaloupe, apples, persimmons, papaya, peaches, strawberries, kelp, nori, figs, mushrooms, radish, swiss chard, and pumpkin	ginger, onions, garlic, fennel, cinnamon, alcohol, and coffee
dry, hacking cough—that annoying cough that just won't go away, even after you're not sick anymore—or lung cancer	lung yin deficiency	nori, kombu, wakame, tofu, miso, pears, apples, oranges, bananas, peaches, strawberries, watermelons, tomatoes, string beans, persimmon, peanuts, and spirulina	onions, leeks, basil, horseradish, cayenne, spicy peppers, ginger, cloves, and cinnamon

Acknowledgments

Kathleen Rushall of Marsal Lyon, Meghan, Joshua, and Mary Norris and my team at Skirt!: I couldn't be luckier to have your support and utter genius. Thanks for believing in me from the very start.

Thanks to Jerome (*mon ami!*), Peter, Michael, Tanya, and Amara for your support, love, patience, creative genius, and amazing works of art. From my very first business card so many years ago to having a gorgeous logo and awesome website, I thank you all.

To all my friends past and present: You all know who you are and how much you mean to me. I'm grateful for your love, kindness, generosity, shared laughter, and lots of vegan deliciousness. Carolyn: Chica, I have endless gratitude to you for sharing your learning curve with me. David, when the words were stuck in my brain, you helped dig them out.

Thanks to my family for your excitement in sharing this dream with me. And a very special thanks goes to Mom and Lee for being my first editors and my biggest fans.

To my teachers and healers along the way: I owe a great debt to all of you for pushing me and helping me to become a better version of myself every day. I wouldn't have had the courage to write this book without you.

To all of my patients: I've learned so much from each and every one of you. Thanks for putting your faith in me, being courageous, and taking this journey with me. I love what I do and have written this book because of you.

To health advocates, TCM practitioners, plant-based nutritionists, and animal lovers everywhere: Your knowledge, compassion, bravery, strength, and perseverance are what keep me going.

To Gyatso, my little man, you taught me patience and unconditional love. I miss you.

Glossary

Acidic having a pH below 7. The more acidic your diet and body, the more prone you will be to illness, inflammation, and injury.

Acupoint acupuncture points.

Acupressure a technique using the same concept of acupoints as acupuncture, but applying slight pressure with the fingers, not needles, to specific pressure points on the body.

Acupuncture the placement of disposable, hair-thin needles into specific points along the body's energy channels, which allows qi (energy) to flow within these meridians or pathways. Stimulating qi flow balances a person to relieve symptoms and eliminate illness.

Acute describes a disease or symptoms of short duration but typically severe.

ADD, ADHD (attention deficit disorder, attention-deficit/hyperactivity disorder) a problem of not being able to focus, being overactive, not being able control behavior, or a combination of these.

Adrenal fatigue a condition in which the adrenal glands are exhausted and unable to produce adequate quantities of hormones, primarily cortisol.

Adrenal glands sit atop the kidneys; responsible for producing cortisol as well as aldosterone, which regulates water levels in the body.

Adrenaline a hormone secreted by the adrenal glands in response to stress.

Aldosterone a corticosteroid hormone released by the adrenal glands that stimulates absorption of sodium by the kidneys and so regulates water and salt balance.

Algae a large group of nonflowering aquatic plants that includes the seaweeds; high in chlorophyll.

Alkaline having a pH above 7; alkaline foods reduce inflammation and prevent disease.

Anemia a condition marked by a deficiency of red blood cells or hemoglobin in the blood, resulting in paleness and weakness.

Antioxidant a substance that inhibits oxidation and protects from disease; found in high levels in most plant foods.

Appendix a sac attached to and opening into the lower end of the large intestine.

Autism/autism spectrum disorders a group of developmental disabilities that can cause significant social, communication, and behavioral challenges.

Autoimmune disease any of a large group of diseases characterized by abnormal functioning of the immune system, causing it to produce antibodies against your own tissues; examples include multiple sclerosis (MS) and lupus.

B-complex originally thought to be a single vitamin but now separated into several B vitamins.

Beta-blockers medication that controls heart rhythm, treats angina, and reduces high blood pressure.

Beta-carotene a compound converted into vitamin A in the liver.

Bile digestive juice secreted by the liver and stored in the gallbladder; aids in the digestion of fats.

Bioenergetics the study of the transformation of energy in living organisms.

Bladder a sac for the temporary retention of urine.

Blood fluid that carries oxygen to and carbon dioxide from the tissues of the body.

Blood deficiency not enough blood in an organ; anemia.

Blood sugar the concentration of glucose in the blood.

Candida an overgrowth of yeast in the digestive tract.

Carbohydrates compounds occurring in foods and living tissues, including sugars, starch, and cellulose.

Celiac disease a disease in which the small intestine is hypersensitive to gluten, leading to difficulty in digesting food containing gluten.

Channels see *meridians*

Chinese herbs customized herbal prescriptions administered in Traditional Chinese Medicine (TCM) based on an individual's symptoms and constitution. Chinese herbal medicine's goal is to treat the source of a problem and eradicate it.

Chronic an illness persisting for a long time or constantly recurring.

Circadian clock/rhythm an internal cyclical process that produces a particular change in a cell or organism within a period of about twenty-four hours; for example, the sleep-wakefulness cycle in humans.

Cleanse the removal of toxins from the body with herbal and/or dietary changes. This can be done through cleansing the liver, the bowel, the blood, and other organs. It is sometimes used in conjunction with fasting.

Congenital a disease present at birth.

Cortisol a hormone released by the adrenal glands in response to stress.

Daiya cheese a vegan, nondairy cheese containing no soy.

Deficiency lack of a particular substance, for example qi, yin, yang, or blood.

Dehydration a depletion or lack of bodily fluids.

Detox/detoxify/detoxing see *cleanse*

Diagnosis identification of an illness by examination of the symptoms.

Digestive enzymes enzymes that break down food to facilitate their absorption by the body.

Diuretic causing increased passing of urine.

Dysmenorrheal menstrual cramps.

ECG (electrocardiogram) an interpretation of the electrical activity of the heart over a period of time, as detected by electrodes attached to the surface of the skin and recorded by a device external to the body.

Eczema a medical condition in which patches of skin become rough and inflamed, with blisters that cause itching and bleeding.

Empath those with the ability to understand and share the feelings of another.

Essential fatty acids (EFAs) fatty acids that humans must ingest because the body requires them for good health but cannot synthesize them.

Estrogen a group of steroid hormones that promote the development and maintenance of female characteristics of the body.

5-element theory the ancient Chinese theory that all living things and all of nature are made up five elements: Wood, Earth, Fire, Metal, and Water.

Flank the side of a person's body between the ribs and the hip

Free radicals unstable molecules that are ferociously searching for their missing electrons and causing untold havoc along the way.

Gallbladder the organ beneath the liver that stores bile after secretion by the liver and before release into the intestines; aids in digestion of fat.

Ginger a hot, fragrant spice that aids in digestion and is used in cooking and drinks, preserved in syrup, or candied.

Ginseng a plant tuber credited with various tonic and medicinal properties.

Gluten a protein found in wheat, rye, barley, and spelt; a common cause of food sensitivities.

Glycemic index a system that ranks foods on a scale from 1 to 100 based on their effect on blood sugar levels.

GMOs (genetically modified organisms) food that has foreign genetic material forced into it to achieve a particular result, like more color, bug resistance, or higher yields.

He Gu acupoint on the hand used for pain, stress, and constipation.

Healing crisis a temporary increase in or flushing out of symptoms during the cleansing or detox process; may be mild or severe.

Heart the organ that pumps blood through the body, traditionally thought to be the seat of emotion.

Heavy metal poisoning the toxic accumulation of heavy metals in the soft tissues of the body.

Herbology the study of herbs and their medical properties.

Hodgkin's disease a type of lymphoma, a cancer originating from white blood cells called lymphocytes.

Holter monitor a portable device that records the rhythm of the heart continuously, typically for twenty-four to forty-eight hours, by means of electrodes attached to the chest.

Hyperkeratosis an abnormal thickening of the outer layer of the skin.

IBS (irritable bowel syndrome) symptoms include abdominal pain, gas, and diarrhea.

Infertility the state of being unable to produce offspring.

Inflammation a physical condition in which part of the body becomes reddened, swollen, hot, and/or often painful; can be the reaction to injury or infection.

Jing qi qi that comes from your ancestors, your genetic inheritance.

Juicing when juice is extracted from vegetables and/or fruit; can be used when doing a cleanse.

Kelp a large brown seaweed with many health benefits.

Kidneys two bean-shaped excretory organs that filter wastes from the blood and excrete them in urine.

Kombu edible kelp that can be used for reducing gas when eating beans and for adding flavor.

Large intestine the second-to-last part of the digestive system that absorbs water from the remaining indigestible food matter and then passes waste material from the body.

LDL (low-density lipoprotein) a form of cholesterol; high levels are associated with increased risk of coronary heart disease and atherosclerosis.

Leaky gut syndrome a medical condition of intestinal or bowel hyperpermeability.

Legumes family of food including beans, peas, peanuts, and lentils.

Liver the organ located in the upper right portion of the abdominal cavity; secretes bile and helps metabolize protein, carbohydrates, and fat; synthesizes substances involved in the clotting of the blood; synthesizes vitamin A; detoxifies poisonous and toxic substances.

Liver enzymes proteins produced by the liver that help speed up chemical reactions such as metabolism, filtration, storage, and excretion.

Lungs a pair of organs situated within the ribcage, into which air is drawn so that oxygen can pass into the blood and carbon dioxide can be removed.

Lymph nodes part of the immune system.

Lymphatic system the interconnected system of spaces and vessels between body tissues and organs by which lymph circulates throughout the body.

Magnesium chemical element that keeps blood pressure normal, bones strong, and regulates the heart rate.

Manganese chemical element that aids in healthy bone structure and metabolism.

Melatonin a hormone secreted by the pineal gland that is connected with regulating the reproductive and sleep cycles.

Menopause the time in a woman's life in which the menstrual cycle ends.

Menorrhagia abnormally heavy bleeding at menstruation.

Meridians set of pathways in the body along which qi flows.

Miso a paste made from fermented soybeans and barley or rice malt; used in traditional Japanese cooking.

MRI (magnetic resonance imaging) a technique that utilizes the properties of magnetic fields to provide images of the body.

Nonorganic/inorganic describes substances that do not derive from organic nature, such as minerals in stones.

Nori an edible seaweed, eaten either fresh or dried in sheets and often used for making vegetable sushi.

Nut butters any ground nuts blended into a butter.

Nutritional yeast a deactivated yeast that is high in B vitamins.

Obese extremely overweight; weighing more than 20 percent (for men) or 25 percent (for women) over their ideal weight determined by height and build.

OCD (obsessive-compulsive disorder) an anxiety disorder in which people have unwanted and repeated thoughts, feelings, ideas, obsessions, or behaviors that make them feel driven to do something.

Omega-3s fatty acids that help lower triglycerides and blood pressure; studies show that omega-3 fatty acids may help with other conditions, including rheumatoid arthritis and depression.

Organic relating to foodstuff that is grown or raised without synthetic fertilizers, antibiotics, pesticides, or hormones.

Oxidation process in which attacks of free radicals, or unstable molecules, subject our cells to continuous damage; also known as oxidative stress.

Pathways see *meridians*

Pericardium tissue surrounding and protecting the heart.

Phosphorous chemical element that aids in healthy bone formation, improved digestion, regulated excretion, protein formation, hormonal balance, and improved energy extraction.

Physiology the branch of biology that deals with the normal functions of living organisms and their parts.

Phytonutrients plant nutrients that increase overall health and protect against certain diseases, including cancer.

Plant-based diet eating a vegan diet that contains no animal products.

PMS premenstrual syndrome; characterized by mood swings, bloating, water retention, low back pain, and/or uterine cramping.

PMSing mood swings and physical discomfort that may occur before menses.

Prebiotics a food source to make probiotic bacteria more effective; some prebiotics enhance the absorption of important minerals like calcium.

Probiotics live bacteria found naturally in the human intestinal tract that can promote or restore a healthy balance of intestinal flora.

Processed food commercially prepared foods that are packaged in boxes, cans, or bags.

Prolapse a slipping forward or down of one of the parts or organs of the body.

Protein substance that builds new cells, maintains tissues, and synthesizes new proteins, making it possible for you to perform basic bodily functions.

PTSD (post-traumatic stress disorder) an anxiety disorder associated with serious traumatic events and characterized by such symptoms as survivor guilt, anxiety, panic attacks, reliving the trauma in dreams, numbness and lack of involvement with reality, or recurrent thoughts and images.

Pungent having a sharp, strong taste or smell.

Qi the energy or life force of the body.

Qi deficiency a lack of qi that is seen with symptoms of fatigue, weakness, and/or low immunity.

Qi stagnation when qi is blocked or not flowing smoothly.

Red blood cells deliver oxygen throughout the body.

Rosacea a condition in which certain facial blood vessels enlarge, giving the face a flushed appearance.

San Jiao "triple burner"; energy system in Chinese medicine that has no equivalent in Western conventional medicine; related to digestion.

Sclera the white outer layer of the eyeball.

Sea vegetables seaweed or vegetables grown in the sea, including some members of the red, brown, and green algae families.

Small intestine the part of the intestine that runs between the stomach and the large intestine, where digestion is completed.

Smoothie a drink including fruit, nuts, seeds, and/or vegetables blended together.

Spleen an abdominal organ involved in the production and removal of blood cells; part of the immune system.

Stomach the principal organ of digestion.

Stress test a test of cardiovascular fitness made by monitoring the heart rate during a period of increasingly strenuous exercise.

Suppress/suppressing consciously or unconsciously inhibiting an unpleasant idea or memory to avoid feeling it.

Tai chi a Chinese system of slow meditative physical exercise designed for relaxation, balance, and health.

Taoism a Chinese philosophy based on the writings of Lao-tzu (sixth century BC), advocating humility and religious piety; means "the Way."

TCM Traditional Chinese Medicine, which is over 5,000 years old and includes healing modalities such as acupuncture, herbal medicine, massage, and nutrition.

Tempeh Indonesian food made by a natural culturing fermentation process that binds soybeans into a cake form; can be used as a meat substitute.

Testosterone a steroid hormone that stimulates development of male secondary sexual characteristics, produced mainly in the testes, but also in the ovaries and adrenal cortex.

Thymus gland generates T lymphocytes, which are white blood cells that help the immune system.

Thyroid gland an organ in the neck that secretes hormones regulating growth and development through the rate of metabolism.

Trauma emotional shock following a stressful event or a physical injury; may be associated with physical shock and sometimes leads to long-term neurosis.

Triglycerides the main constituents of natural fats and oils; high concentrations in the blood indicate an elevated risk of stroke.

Tryptophan helps metabolize protein, improve sleep quality, elevate your mood.

Turmeric bright yellow aromatic plant of the ginger family, used for several healing properties such as boosting the immune system and muscle pain, and also for flavoring and coloring in Asian cooking and formerly as a fabric dye.

Vegan a person who does not eat, wear, or use any animal products; the term can relate to just diet where no animal products are consumed.

Vegenaise a vegan version of mayonnaise made by Follow Your Heart.

Vertebrae the series of small bones forming the spine, having several projections for articulation and muscle attachment, and a hole through which the spinal cord passes.

Vitamix a professional-grade blender, excellent for making pureed soups, nut butters, and smoothies.

Western medicine system in which doctors and other health-care professionals (such as nurses, pharmacists, and therapists) treat symptoms and diseases using drugs, radiation, or surgery; also called conventional medicine, mainstream medicine, orthodox medicine, biomedicine, and allopathic medicine.

White blood cells part of the immune system used to defend the body against the infection.

Whole foods foods that are unprocessed and unrefined before being consumed.

Yang the active male principle of the universe, characterized as creative and associated with heaven, heat, and light; based in Taoism.

Yang deficiency a lack of yang, often characterized by symptoms being worse during the day; may display as feeling cold.

Yellow Emperor's Classic of Medicine the most important ancient text on Chinese medicine, written in approximately 500 BC.

Yin the passive female principle of the universe, characterized as sustaining and associated with Earth, dark, and cold; originates from Taoism.

Yin deficiency a lack of yin, often characterized by symptoms increasing at night; may manifest as feeling hot.

Yin Tang acupoint between the eyebrows for calming and sedating.

Index

About the Author

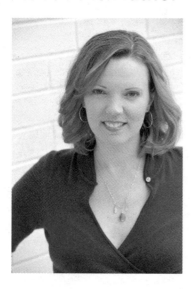

Heather Lounsbury, L.Ac., one of Los Angeles's best-known acupuncturists, is the powerhouse behind the *Live Natural. Live Well* brand, embracing a popular blog, YouTube videos, and weekly radio show. She has attracted broad media attention from *Time, Billboard* magazine, Fox News, *Business Week,* and *VegNews,* among others. She is passionate about spreading the message of holistic living and empowering her patients to heal themselves. She lives in Santa Monica, California. Visit her at LiveNaturalLiveWell.com.